Instructor's Manual to Accompany

Respiratory Care:

A GUIDE TO CLINICAL PRACTICE, FOURTH EDITION

Instructor's Manual to Accompany

Respiratory Care:

A GUIDE TO CLINICAL PRACTICE

FOURTH EDITION

Mark Simmons, MSEd, RRT, RPFT
Program Director
York College, York Hospital
School of Respiratory Therapy
York, Pennsylvania

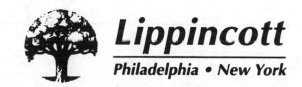

Lippincott
Philadelphia • New York

Acquisitions Editor: Lawrence McGrew
Coordinating Editorial Assistant: Holly Collins
Ancillary Editor: Doris S. Wray
Project Editor: Gretchen Metzger
Production Manager: Helen Ewan
Production Coordinator: Nannette Winski
Design Coordinator: Doug Smock
Compositor: Pine Tree Composition, Inc.
Printer/Binder: Victor

6 5 4 3 2 1

ISBN: 0-397-55772-8

Preface

PURPOSE

The instructor's manual for *Respiratory Care: A Guide to Clinical Practice, Fourth Edition* is designed to provide instructors with materials to assist in the teaching and testing of their students. A variety of methods will be utilized to accomplish this task.

ORGANIZATION

In general, the dissemination of information (what we call education) falls into three categories: the "need to know," the "nice to know," and the "nuts to know."

1. The NEED TO KNOW information is the most important. You need this information to perform you job, because it is what an employer will expect new graduates to know. It will also help graduates pass the NBRC exams.
2. The NICE TO KNOW information is next in importance. You can still perform your job satisfactorily without it, but if you want to be an outstanding student or employee you will strive to learn this information.
3. The NUTS TO KNOW information is least important. It can literally be interpreted as, *you are nuts if you know it.* This information has little bearing on whether or not you can do your job properly. But, if you want to be on a sputum bowl quiz team, you should spend some time studying it. On the other hand, I think a liberal arts education is very important (and so do most colleges). Some of the "nuts to know" information, although not job specific, helps to mold us into a better person.

Of course everyone has a different idea of what should be included in each of these categories, so consistency in education can be a problem. Interpreting what is important and what is not, is difficult. This is a chronic problem for educators who need to present the newest and latest information. We have a difficult time finding room for new material in a course because we do not know what we can possibly drop from the course.

With the previous information in mind, you will find that some of the chapters in the instructor's manual will differ radically from others in their content and style. The manual contains 36 chapters, each corresponding to a chapter in *Respiratory Care.* Items that may appear in chapters include:

> Chapter Outline
> Objectives
> Chapter Overview
> Lab Exercises
> Calculation Exercises
> Case Studies
> Test Questions

Due to the diverse nature of the material presented in *Respiratory Care,* from equipment to disease states, from health care reengineering to infection control, not all items will appear in all chapters. I realize that this text will be used for different levels of instruction. I hope that the materials provided will be applicable to your setting. Education should be fun. I hope you can enjoy using the Instructor's Manual while you, and the students, learn.

Acknowledgment

A special thank you to the following individuals for their help in gathering information for some of the case studies presented.

Ann Daugherty
Dave Fillman
Bridgette Flickinger
Jim Heindel
Susan Zimmerman

Mark Simmons, MSEd, RRT, RPFT

Contents

SECTION I

THE RESPIRATORY CARE PROFESSION: PAST, PRESENT, AND FUTURE

1

Roots of the Respiratory Care Profession

History is important to each of us. It is exciting to know from whence we came as we move forward. Unfortunately (or fortunately, depending on your perspective), the National Board for Respiratory Care (NBRC) no longer tests for this knowledge on the credentialing examinations. Because of this, many schools spend little time reviewing the history of the respiratory care profession. With this in mind, have fun and use the following activities to help you review the history of the respiratory care profession as presented in *Respiratory Care*.

WORD FIND

Find the following names, words, and abbreviations in the word find. Words may be horizontal, vertical, or diagonal. They may also be forward or backward.

AARC
Albertus Magnus
Amedeo Avogadro
black death
Boothby
Bulbulian
CPAP
Drager
ECMO
Elisha
Forrest Bird
Gay Lussac
Hasselbalch
Henderson
IPPB
IVOX

Jack Emerson
Jacques Charles
John Haldane
JRCRTE
Lovelace
Maimonides
Moses
NBRC
Paul Bert
Ray Bennett
Reynolds
Roger Bacon
Thomas Petty
William Henry
Yersinia pestis

A	P	N	G	N	U	S	B	O	Y	L	D	I	S	S	E	H	O	E	K	P	O	C	S
C	R	A	A	W	V	O	P	L	L	O	O	K	I	T	T	E	V	I	S	E	R	U	E
R	V	I	C	E	O	R	P	O	A	P	J	A	C	K	E	M	E	R	S	O	N	R	N
I	F	L	O	T	X	D	I	T	E	C	E	F	A	A	T	I	N	I	M	G	O	A	A
E	R	U	H	G	O	O	D	L	U	C	K	I	D	I	W	N	S	K	A	A	C	N	D
L	E	B	R	L	A	K	V	I	N	O	O	D	O	R	U	O	E	M	D	Y	A	R	L
L	Y	L	U	L	V	R	A	Y	B	E	N	N	E	T	T	Q	S	I	A	L	B	O	A
I	N	U	Q	E	O	H	I	E	R	A	E	W	A	A	E	U	U	K	F	U	R	B	H
J	O	B	A	B	G	A	N	L	C	O	T	H	N	D	T	O	O	E	Q	S	E	L	N
S	L	A	E	Z	A	S	N	I	C	E	W	H	S	R	A	H	H	J	I	S	G	A	H
T	D	C	V	E	G	S	A	J	F	I	B	O	E	L	I	S	H	A	N	A	O	R	O
H	S	K	A	L	R	E	T	A	L	L	A	B	D	N	E	A	R	C	U	C	R	K	J
O	R	I	C	L	O	L	U	L	A	U	L	G	I	N	D	N	I	Q	O	T	S	E	A
M	O	F	I	N	W	B	I	B	L	A	X	I	N	O	T	E	X	U	T	I	E	V	R
A	M	E	D	E	O	A	V	O	G	A	D	R	O	A	D	K	R	E	R	T	T	E	S
S	O	T	H	I	M	L	O	O	P	A	R	E	M	R	O	A	A	S	R	T	N	E	T
P	U	T	Y	H	I	C	O	U	A	Y	I	V	I	N	E	T	T	C	O	T	T	X	N
E	Q	O	E	X	L	H	S	Q	U	I	C	P	A	P	O	G	R	H	E	N	A	A	N
T	R	N	N	O	B	O	R	N	L	N	A	E	M	A	T	J	A	A	N	I	L	L	O
T	R	I	L	V	I	N	N	E	B	D	R	I	B	T	S	E	R	R	O	F	E	S	J
Y	E	R	S	I	N	I	A	P	E	S	T	I	S	O	I	P	I	L	D	E	C	S	A
A	N	N	E	T	T	E	N	S	R	U	S	T	O	L	H	A	Z	E	Z	A	M	O	T
G	E	C	A	L	E	V	O	L	T	O	V	R	B	E	Z	P	I	S	E	S	O	M	E

CROSSWORD PUZZLE

Each of the following clues will be answered by the last name of the individual involved. In some cases, a single name is given; therefore, that name is used. Each of the answers can be found in Respiratory Care.

Down
1. world spirit
2. phlegm
3. father of inhalation therapy
4. oxygen electrode
5. burned at stake
6. ear oximeter
7. auscultation
8. spirometer
9. syphilis
10. streptomycin

Across
1. pulse oximetry
2. altitude
3. oxygen tents
4. pneumatic theory
5. AMBU
6. philosophical transactions
7. heart muscular pump
8. fireplace bellows
9. rabies
10. cardiac output
11. oxygen content
12. ether
13. carbon dioxide electrode

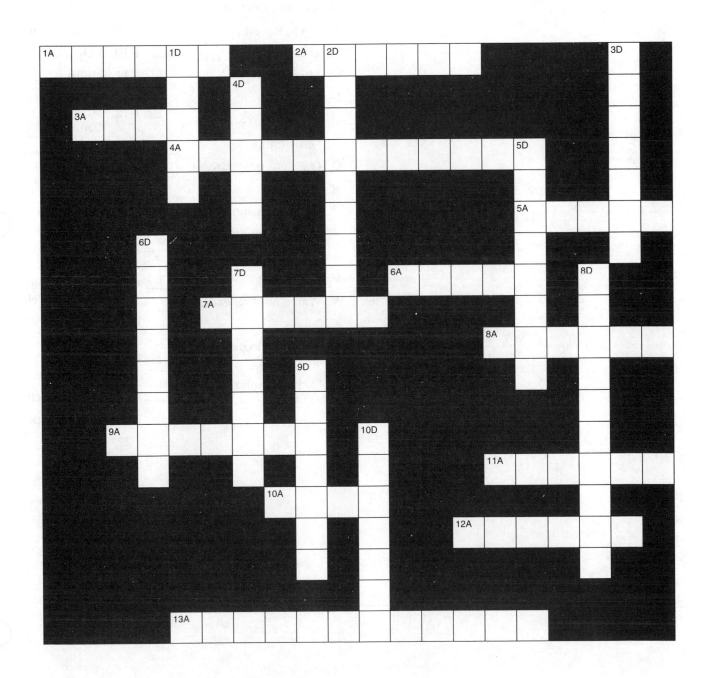

MATCHING

Place the appropriate letter of the left hand column on the line in the right hand column that best matches. Each letter will be used only one time. Answers can be found in Respiratory Care.

A. Atomic theory

B. Barometer

C. Carbon dioxide

D. Decapitated

E. Essential humor

F. Fire air

G. Gas therapy with tents

H. Human dissection

I. Iron lung

J. Jackson, Chevalier

K. Koch, Robert

L. Laughing gas

M. Microscope

N. Nursing

O. Oxygen curve

P. Penicillium

Q. Quotient (respiratory)

R. Red Cross

S. Surface tension

T. Tracheal Intubation

U. Used cannula therapy

V. Venti mask

W. Water, air, fire, earth

X. X-rays

Y. Ye ole "Phlogisticated air"

Z. Lazzaro Spallazani

_____ 1-1. Joseph Black

_____ 1-2. Carl Scheele

_____ 1-3. Alexander Fleming

_____ 1-4. Ivan Magill

_____ 1-5. John Dalton

_____ 1-6. Florence Nightingale

_____ 1-7. Christian Bohr

_____ 1-8. William Roentgen

_____ 1-9. Clara Barton

_____ 1-10. VO_2, VCO_2

_____ 1-11. Philip Drinker

_____ 1-12. Morgan Campbell

_____ 1-13. Pythagoras

_____ 1-14. Leonardo da Vinci

_____ 1-15. Evangelista Torricelli

_____ 1-16. Antoine Lavoisier

_____ 1-17. Anthony van Leeuwenhoek

_____ 1-18. Gardner Colton

_____ 1-19. Joseph Priestley

_____ 1-20. Alvan Barach

_____ 1-21. laryngoscope

_____ 1-22. T.B.

_____ 1-23. Eduard Pfluger

_____ 1-24. Pierre Simon de Laplace

_____ 1-25. Hippocrates

_____ 1-26. Sir Arbuthnot Lane

2

Respiratory Care in the 1990s

REVIEW QUESTIONS

2-1. Which of the following is true concerning open-ended questions during a patient interview?
A. they are always written
B. they can be answered with a "yes" or "no"
C. they allow in-depth responses
D. they are inappropriate for an interview

2-2. Encoding is defined as:
A. communicating using computers
B. the use of technical jargon
C. communication without speech
D. the transforming of ideas into symbols

2-3. The "captain of the ship" in the respiratory care profession has historically been recognized as the:
A. physician
B. respiratory care administrator
C. respiratory care department director
D. respiratory care supervisor

2-4. The respiratory profession's credentialing arm for practitioners is the:
A. AARC
B. BOMA
C. NBRC
D. JRCRTE

2-5. Health care currently consumes what percent of the gross national product?
A. 8%
B. 13%
C. 19%
D. 24%

2-6. The number of Americans with no health care coverage is estimated to be:
A. 10 million
B. 20 million
C. 30 million
D. 40 million

2-7. Approximately what percent of workers say that work is the main source of stress in their lives?
A. 20%
B. 30%
C. 50%
D. 80%

2-8. Which of the following refer to change driven by crises?
I. externally motivated
II. internally driven
III. reactive
IV. proactive

A. I and III
B. I and IV
C. II and III
D. II and IV

2-9. When considering reengineering through automation, CPR stands for:
A. complete pulmonary rehabilitation
B. cardiopulmonary resuscitation
C. competent personnel revisited
D. computerized patient record

2-10. At the turn of the century (1900), most health care was delivered where?
A. the home
B. skilled nursing facility
C. subacute facility
D. long-term facility

2-11. The reemergence of home care is a result of each of the following except:
A. cost-containment pressures
B. consumer preferences
C. physician preferences
D. new technologies

2-12. The goal of communication is to:
A. send and receive messages
B. create understanding
C. share information
D. interpret body language

2-13. All of the following are true concerning therapist-driven protocols (TDPs) except:
A. physicians must order TDPs to have them started
B. physicians may override TDPs
C. physicians may discontinue TDPs
D. good TDP orders have no boundaries

2-14. Each of the following are true concerning "duty of care" except:
   A. this physician-patient relationship is the basis of all medical practice
   B. this agreement can be viewed as a contractual or professional one
   C. this relationship can be terminated by the patient at any time
   D. this relationship can be terminated by the physician at any time

2-15. The most frequent reason for litigation between patient and physician is:
   A. negligence
   B. invasion of privacy
   C. fraud
   D. breach of confidentiality

2-16. For patient consent to be legally meaningful, it must meet each of the following criteria except:
   A. written down
   B. given by a person legally entitled to do so
   C. freely given
   D. informed consent

3

The Future of the Respiratory Care Profession

It is uncertain what changes the next years will bring to the health care industry. As respiratory care professionals, we are concerned not only about the industry but also about what these changes will mean to us specifically. We need to be flexible and willing to change to meet the challenges that we will face. I think we need to consider the words of Thomas Henry Huxley: "The rung of a ladder was never meant to rest upon but only to hold a man's foot long enough to enable him to put the other somewhat higher."

Although I do not think our profession has been resting, I think it is time to move on to keep pace with or, more importantly, keep ahead of change. In the process of change, many new and confusing terms and processes have been introduced into the health care system. I would like to review some of these.

KEY TERMS AND DEFINITIONS

Third-party payers: A third-party payer refers to employers, insurance companies, the government, and others who pay for a patient's medical bill.

Fee-For-Service, also know as Indemnity: In this process, providers (health care facilities, physicians, and others) charge a fee for every service or therapy provided to a patient. Although helping to promote industry growth, many consider it a factor that contributes to the high cost of health care.

Alternative Delivery System: A phrase referring to all other payment programs except fee-for-service.

Diagnosis-Related Group (DRG) and Prospective Payment System (PPS): To try to help reduce governmental costs for health care, Medicare changed its reimbursement system to one based on patient diagnosis. Providers were given a set amount of money or flat rate to care for a patient based on the patient's diagnosis. *Example:* Let's say that the DRG reimbursement for a patient with pneumonia is set at $10,000. If the hospital is able to treat the patient for a cost of $8,000 instead of $10,000, the difference of $2,000 is a profit for the hospital. On the other hand, if the hospital spends $12,000 treating the patient, they lose $2,000 and need to recoup their loses elsewhere.

Managed Care: A philosophy and broad term used to describe (1) organizations that combine the finances and delivery of health care services (HMO, PPO) and (2) the techniques used to control the cost of use of medical services (use review, prior authorization, capitation). This process was designed to improve resource utilization and match the resources with demand. In short, it will most likely result in a rationing of services. An example of this process would involve a company contracting with a provider to deliver the needed health care services its employees may require. Often a set amount of money would be paid whether or not the services are used.

Integrated Delivery Systems: It is the system formed when two or more providers of the health care system join together to deliver health care. The systems incorporate what is known as a continuum of care, including areas such as primary care, ambulatory care, emergency care, acute care, post-acute care, home care, and custodial care. Only time will tell if some of these marriages of different varieties of providers will last.

Health Maintenance Organizations (HMOs), Preferred Provider Organizations (PPOs), and Point of Service (POS) Plans: These organizations require that enrollees pay a set annual fee and then receive their care by a single provider or pre-approved providers. A client must often be evaluated by a primary care physician or gatekeeper before seeing a specialist or visiting a hospital, unless it is an emergency. These organizations use the philosophy of managed care. Some of the organizations are more strict than others in their requirements. It is often normal to have a co-payment for medical service rendered, and use of providers outside the network results in increased expense for the enrollee.

Capitation: Unlike fee-for-service where a fee is paid for each service rendered, capitation limits the amount of payment to a provider. It is a technique used by managed care to control costs. In this system, there is a cap or limited amount of money received by the provider for each patient it treats. It is in the interest of the provider to appropriately treat the patient, but to do it with the least number of services and at the lowest cost. Remember that, although the hospital is trying to reduce its costs, it is still expected to retain a high quality of care. *Example:* Business A has 100 employees. Business A contracts with Community Hospital to provide all the health care needs of business A employees. The hospital agrees to accept $1,000/year/employee to deliver this care or a total of $100,000 for the year. Over the year it cost the Hospital $80,000 for care of the employees of business A. The hospital made a profit of $20,000. The following year the contract was again renewed for the same amount. This time, however, one of the employees needed open heart surgery and another was involved in a motor vehicle accident with extensive trauma. The cost of care was $150,000 for this year, and the hospital was set back $50,000.

To remain competitive, hospitals need to reduce their overall expenses as much as possible. Managed care and capitation have forced hospitals into *reengineering* (or *restructuring* or *reorganization*).[1] This means hospitals will do away with all nonessential services to help preserve a bottom line with a positive balance. It is also forcing providers to reconsider where and how care is given. This is leading to the growth of alternate sites for health care (any place outside the hospital) where overall costs are less.

Patient-Focused Care: Patient-focused care is a facet of hospital reorganization where health care workers are no longer assigned to a specific department (eg, Respiratory Care, ECG). These departments will be decentralized and workers will be assigned to a multidisciplinary team that is responsible for a given area of the hospital (ie, a given number of patient beds). This type of care will attempt to bring as many of the services to the patient's bedside as possible. This system is intended to decrease costs and increase efficiency.

Multiskilling: Multiskilling or cross-training ties in with patient-focused care. It is a process where individuals are taught to perform numerous tasks. In this scenario, one person will take the place of numerous other workers. The skills these individuals will be taught, finding instructors to teach them, and the role of credentialing and state licensure in this process are yet to be seen.

AARC Clinical Practice Guidelines (CPGs): CPGs are statements developed to assist practitioners in the delivery of appropriate respiratory care and to improve the quality of that care. The use of the guidelines may also help to control costs, improve outcomes, and increase patient satisfaction.

Protocols (Therapist Guided, Patient Driven): Statements or flow charts used to guide practitioners in the delivery of appropriate care for a given patient situation. These are institution specific. CPGs may be useful in the development of protocols.

Clinical Pathways: A clinical or critical pathway is a process that monitors and facilitates the coordination of average patient care through the use of a standardized, interdisciplinary process. Patient interventions, such as tests, therapies, teaching, and discharge planning, are sequenced based on time or outcomes. The desire is to achieve specific goals and results (patient outcomes) within a specific time period.

Demand Management (DM) or Demand Engineering: DM focuses on patients and not providers. The goal of DM is to decrease the demand for health care services by controlling utilization. Reductions must target inappropriate or unnecessary care. A main component of DM is *disease management*. Disease management has its emphasis on preventing disease or managing it aggressively when intervention will have its greatest impact. Two concepts lie at the heart of disease management. First, it involves public education so that people know when to seek medical care. Second, it involves the development of standardized treatments for specific diseases, especially chronic diseases, with the involvement of patients in their own plan. In reality, it is a combination of patient/public education, clinical pathways, and case management covering *all* aspects of patient care in *any* patient care setting.

Does the average practitioner need to understand all of this information to perform his or her job? Will students be tested on this information on the national examinations? The answer is no to both of these questions, but this information affects each of us, and we need to know what is happening in the health care setting.

---

[1]The latest buzz words and terms are a dime a dozen (even with inflation) and are constantly changing. It becomes a little frustrating when there seems to be no good reason for much of the change. This is just one example that can be found many times in the literature. By the time this study guide is published, some of the terms will have changed again.

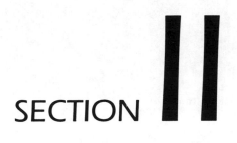

SECTION II

RESPIRATORY GAS EXCHANGE MECHANISMS

4

The Anatomical Basis for Respiratory Gas Exchange

REVIEW QUESTIONS

4-1. The primary function of the human lung is to:
   A. act as a blood reservoir
   B. serve as a filter
   C. allow gas exchange
   D. transform biochemical compounds

4-2. Internal respiration is:
   A. the same as ventilation (V_T exchange)
   B. the movement of oxygen into and carbon dioxide out of the cell
   C. the diffusion of gas from the lung
   D. the same as adenosine triphosphate production

4-3. Particulate matter greater than how many micrometers is filtered in the nose?
   A. 1 μm
   B. 3 μm
   C. 5 μm
   D. 10 μm

4-4. The sensory receptors for olfactory nerves are located near which of the following?
   A. superior turbinate
   B. middle turbinate
   C. inferior turbinate
   D. inferior meatus

4-5. Which of the following is a paired cartilage?
   A. thyroid
   B. arytenoid
   C. epiglottis
   D. cricoid

4-6. The Adam's Apple refers to which cartilage?
   A. cuneiform
   B. epiglottic
   C. thyroid
   D. cricoid

4-7. The vesicular folds are also called the:
   A. true vocal folds
   B. false vocal folds
   C. glottis
   D. vocal ligaments

4-8. Cartilage is present in airways until which airway level?
   A. segmental bronchi
   B. subsegmental bronchi
   C. terminal bronchioles
   D. respiratory bronchioles

4-9. Approximately what percent of total airway flow resistance is caused by gas flow in the bronchioles?
   A. 80%
   B. 60%
   C. 40%
   D. 20%

4-10. Which cell type forms the majority of the alveolar cellular lining?
   A. type I
   B. type II
   C. type III
   D. Clara cells

4-11. The interalveolar communications that allow collateral movement of air are the:
   A. channels of Martin
   B. canals of Lambert
   C. pores of Kohn

4-12. Alveoli, which are first seen in the fetus, will increase in number until what age?
   A. 1 month following birth
   B. 1 year of age
   C. 2 years of age
   D. 8 years of age

4-13. According to the law of Laplace, for a given surface tension, as radius decreases, the pressure required to keep a sphere from collapsing will:
   A. increase
   B. decrease
   C. not be affected

4-14. Normally at rest, less than what percent of total oxygen consumption is used by the respiratory muscles?
   A. 50%
   B. 30%
   C. 10%
   D. 5%

4-15. The medullary chemoreceptors are influenced primarily by which factor?
   A. CSF PO_2
   B. CSF PCO_2
   C. CSF pH
   D. arterial oxygen

4-16. In the upright position, the $\dot{V}/\dot{Q}$ is highest in which part of the lung?
  A. upper lung (independent)
  B. mid lung
  C. lower lung (dependent)

4-17. The most common cause of hypoxemia is:
  A. true shunt
  B. $\dot{V}/\dot{Q}$ mismatch
  C. hypoventilation
  D. diffusion defects

5

The Physicochemical Basis for Respiratory Gas Exchange

REVIEW QUESTIONS

5-1. Using equation 1 in Equation Box 5-1 in *Respiratory Care*, what is the PaO_2 when PB = 760 mmHg, FiO_2 = 0.21, $PaCO_2$ = 40 mmHg, and R – 0.8?
   A. 82 mmHg
   B. 92 mmHg
   C. 102 mmHg
   D. 112 mmHg

5-2. Using equation 1 in Equation Box 5-1 in *Respiratory Care*, what is the PAO_2 when PB = 680 mmHg, FiO_2 = 0.40, $PACO_2$ = 50 mmHg, and R = 0.7?
   A. 160 mmHg
   B. 170 mmHg
   C. 180 mmHg
   D. 190 mmHg

5-3. Oxygen passes from the alveoli to the blood by:
   A. active transport
   B. osmosis
   C. diffusion
   D. ion channels

5-4. Blood flowing to the tissues has its oxyhemoglobin curve shifted to the right because of:
   A. decreased CO_2
   B. decreased temperature
   C. decreased 2,3-diphosphoglycerate
   D. decreased pH

5-5. Normal P_{50} is:
   A. 26.5 mmHg
   B. 37 mmHg
   C. 44 mmHg
   D. 47 mmHg

5-6. One gram of hemoglobin can carry how much oxygen when 100% saturated?
   A. 1.21 mL
   B. 1.38 mL
   C. 1.34 mL
   D. 1.43 mL

5-7. A mild but low $\dot{V}/\dot{Q}$ will most likely result in which of the following?
   A. decreased pH
   B. increased $PaCO_2$
   C. increased HCO_3
   D. decreased PaO_2

5-8. Which of the following formulas is appropriate to calculate oxygen delivery?
   A. cardiac output × hemoglobin level
   B. cardiac output × oxygen content
   C. oxygen content × total blood volume
   D. PaO_2 × 1.34

5-9. Lack of oxygen in body tissue is signaled by the production of which of the following?
   A. HCO_3
   B. a volatile acid
   C. lactic acid
   D. adenosine triphosphate

5-10. Carbohydrate utilization in metabolism is indicated by an exchange ratio of:
   A. 0.7
   B. 0.8
   C. 0.9
   D. 1.0

SECTION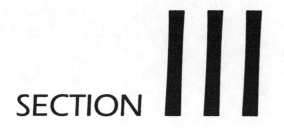

CLINICAL ASSESSMENT OF CARDIOPULMONARY FUNCTION

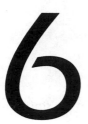

6

Assessment Skills Core to Practitioner Success

Currently, many respiratory care practitioners (RCPs) are limited in their ability to apply all of the formal assessment skills presented in *Respiratory Care*. This is because many of the RCPs are expected to perform many duties (treatments) in a finite time period, thus they do not have the time to perform long assessments. Historically, most of the extensive patient assessments were, and are, routinely performed by other health care personnel (physicians, physician assistants, and nurse practitioners). Hopefully, RCPs have time to briefly scan patient reports before administering treatments. With the revamping of the health care industry, the role of the RCP is changing. Assessment is becoming, and will continue to become, a more important role for the RCP. It is imperative that students make good use of their clinical time and become much more proficient in their ability to assess patients.

RESPIRATORY ASSESSMENT

Respiratory assessment should involve five different areas including the following:

1. patient history
2. patient interview
3. a physical examination
4. collection of laboratory data
5. a systematic recording method

Patient History

Currently, formal histories are taken by other personnel. The RCP should strive to read this information before patient interaction.

Patient Interview

As with patient histories, formal patient interviews are also done by others. RCPs will often be involved in informal interviews as they interact with patients. These informal times often may be revealing and offer some very good insights about the patient.

Physical Examination

Once again, the RCP often relies on others for much of these data. Of the **vital signs**, pulse rate and respiratory rate are commonly and repeatedly assessed by the RCP. The extent of examination of the chest and lungs by RCPs will vary. Most of the facets of **inspection** should routinely be performed. These include breathing pattern, chest configuration, cough, sputum production, skin color, digital clubbing, edema, and signs of distress. My guess is that **palpation** is a lost art with many RCPs (although many of us never had it to lose). We often rely on the chest radiograph and other sources and procedures to obtain the needed data instead of touching the chest. Of course, few can resist the urge to push on crepitus tissue, especially when showing it to someone for the first time. **Percussion** is likewise an under-used assessment skill and had been abandoned by many. We again rely on the chest radiograph for much of the information we need. The last part of the physical examination, **auscultation**, should be one of the assessment skills used by all RCPs. It is important to be able to distinguish between normal (vesicular) and abnormal (adventitious) breath sounds and to determine between presence and absence of air movement. The evaluation of vocal resonance falls into the "nice to know" arena; this area has been replaced by the chest radiograph and as an assessment skill is waning in its use. This does not mean you should not use the technique. Do not be afraid to ask your patients to perform these techniques. In the long run, both you and your patient will benefit.

Data Collection

Laboratory data is very valuable for a proper assessment. It will be necessary to learn about each of the following. These areas are introduced in Chapter 6 of *Respiratory Care*, and many are discussed in greater detail in subsequent chapters.

Radiologic findings
Sputum evaluation
Pulmonary Function Tests (PFTs)
Arterial blood gases (ABGs)

Oxygen transport studies

Skin testing

Bronchoscopy

Pleural fluid evaluation

Electrocardiograms

Hemodynamics

Hematology, blood chemistry, and electrolytes

Histology and cytology

Documentation of Findings

Some health care practitioners write care plans without the formal SOAP note. For others, the SOAP note is a popular method for recording information on patients while allowing evaluation and planning for the therapy to be initiated. I think the use of the SOAP will help those just beginning to perform care plans to better organize their information.

S = Subjective—what the patient tells you

O = Objective—measured data

A = Assessment—your evaluation of the situation

P = Plan—your proposed plan of therapy for the patient

The SOAP note should *not* be thought of as a once and done activity. It should be carried out every time a patient is treated. It is an ongoing continuous process of obtaining feedback, reevaluating the patient, and updating the treatment plan. The reevaluation process should continue until your services are no longer required.

Students should not become frustrated because they feel overwhelmed. It takes time and a lot of practice to perform an assessment properly. Tell them to hang in there.

From the following information write a short SOAP note on each of these patients.

CASE STUDY 1

History of Present Illness

A 35-year-old white woman is admitted to the emergency department. She states that she experienced sharp pain in her right chest and shortness of breath while carrying a bag of groceries. The pain was sudden in onset, got worse with breathing, and got better when she held her breath. It radiated through to her back, but not to the arm, shoulder, or jaw. It did not change with position or exercise. The patient denied environmental allergies and history of asthma. There was no associated cough, sputum production, fever, night sweats, or orthopnea.

Medical History

Occupation: Homemaker

Marital status: Married with two children

Pets: One house cat

Travel: To Bermuda 2 months ago

Medications: Has been taking Augmentin for sinus infection for 7 days

Smoking history: Has never smoked

Previous illnesses: Usual childhood illnesses

Surgeries: Tonsillectomy at age 10 years, C-section at age 28 years

Family illnesses: Mother has asthma

Physical Examination

General: The patient is a slender, well-developed, well-nourished white woman who appears her stated age. She is alert, oriented, and in moderate respiratory distress during the physical examination.

Vital signs: Within normal limits except for sinus tachycardia at 110.

Head, eyes, ears, nose, and throat (HEENT): No contributing findings.

Neck: The trachea is mildly deviated toward the left. There is no lymphadenopathy, jugular venous distention, or carotid bruit.

Chest: The chest is asymmetrical with more movement on the left side during respiration. Percussion reveals hyper-resonance in the right upper chest.

Lungs: Normal breath sounds on the left; diminished breath sounds in the right upper lobe.

Abdomen: Bowel sounds present, abdomen soft and nontender to palpation. No organomegaly.

Extremities: No cyanosis, clubbing, or edema. Pulses are +2 in all areas.

Chest radiograph: Partial pneumothorax of right lung. Mediastinal shift to the left.

6-1. Write a SOAP note:

S _____

_____

_____

O _____

_____

_____

A _____

_____

_____

P _____

_____

_____

CASE STUDY 2

History of Present Illness

A 64-year-old homeless man is admitted to the emergency department with a 2-day history of cough, shaking chills, and thick, yellow sputum production. The patient is also complaining of moderate dyspnea and pain in the left lower chest area during inspiration. The patient states that he has had no appetite for the last day.

Medical History

Occupation: None
Marital status: Divorced
Pets: One cat
Travel: None in the past 10 years
Medications: None
Smoking history: 40 packs/year
Previous illnesses: Emphysema for 10 years, congestive heart failure for 6 years
Surgeries: Surgery to remove skin cancer 2 years ago
Family illnesses: Unknown

Physical Examination

General: The patient is a poorly nourished, unkempt white man who appears older than his stated age. Patient is alert, oriented, and in severe respiratory distress during the physical examination.

Vital signs: Temperature 38.7°C, sinus tachycardia at 126, respirations 28/min, blood pressure 154/96.

HEENT: No contributing findings.

Neck: The trachea is midline. There is no lymphadenopathy. Mild jugular venous distention is present. There is no carotid bruit.

Chest: Anterior diameter is equal to posterior diameter. Chest expansion is symmetrical. Normal resonance to percussion over most of the chest except the right lower chest, which has decreased resonance.

Lungs: Breath sounds diminished with scattered high-pitched wheezes throughout all lung fields. Fine crackles in right lower lobe. Course rhonchi and bronchial breath sounds in left lower lobe.

Abdomen: Bowel sounds present, abdomen soft and nontender to palpation. No organomegaly.

Extremities: Nail-bed cyanosis of fingers. No clubbing. +1 pitting edema of ankles. Pulses are +2 in all areas except for dorsalis pedis pulses which are +1.

Chest radiograph: Changes consistent with emphysema are noted. Consolidation of right lower lobe consistent with lobar pneumonia.

6-2. Write a SOAP note:

S _____

_____

_____

O _____

_____

_____

A _____

_____

_____

P _____

_____

_____

LABORATORY SKILL—ROLE PLAY

Using a classmate as a patient, have students practice performing a respiratory assessment. Develop a pool of patient situations by writing a diagnosis and appropriate laboratory data on slips of paper and placing them in a container. Have the "patient" pull from the container a patient situation, including the laboratory data, so the "patient" knows how to act and respond to the assessor. Do not allow the assessor to see this information.

A. Practice interviewing and obtain a history on your patient.
  1. Use various types of questions and responses as described in *Respiratory Care*.
  2. Have an observer critique your verbal and nonverbal skills during the interview.
B. Perform a physical examination as outlined in *Respiratory Care*.
  1. Measure vital signs.
  2. Identify thoracic landmarks and inspect the chest noting the following:
     Symmetry of movement
     Tracheal deviation
     Retractions
     Shape of the chest
  3. Note each of the following:
     Ability to cough
     Sputum production: amount and color
     Skin and mucus membrane coloration
     Presence of digital clubbing
     Presence of edema
  4. Palpate the chest noting the following:
     Chest excursion—place thumbs along each costal margin at the back, slide hands medially to raise loose skinfolds between thumbs, ask patient to inhale deeply, note range and symmetry.
     Tactile fremitus—use bony part of palm at base of fingers to palpate vibrations to chest wall when patient speaks. Ask patient to repeat "ninety-nine" or "one-one-one." Vibrations are decreased when lung tissue is consolidated.
  5. Percuss the chest.
     Note percussion sounds
     Determine diaphragm excursion—ask patient to take a deep breath and hold it, percuss up from the lower torso, note area where dullness changes to resonance, mark a line, ask patient to exhale and hold it, percuss till resonance is again noted, mark a line, normal excursion is 3 to 5 cm.
  6. Auscultate the chest.
     Listen for normal and abnormal breath sounds as described in *Respiratory Care*

C. Have the "patient" hand the assessor the clinical data to be evaluated. (This is the prearranged data pulled from the hat.)
D. Write a SOAP note on your findings. (See if your evaluation matches the patient situation pulled from the hat.)

REVIEW QUESTIONS

6-4. During a patient interview, all of the following are appropriate except:
  A. privacy
  B. minimal interruptions
  C. interviewer does most of the talking
  D. comfortable environment
6-5. All of the following are classified as vital signs except:
  A. body temperature
  B. urine output
  C. blood pressure
  D. respiratory rate
6-6. A patient with a change of temperature from 37.0°C in the morning to 37.5°C in the evening has:
  A. hypothermia
  B. a definite fever
  C. a definite bacterial infection
  D. a normal diurnal variation in temperature
6-7. Which of the following would most likely affect oral temperature readings?
  A. nasal cannula
  B. simple mask
  C. air-entrainment mask
  D. cool-mist aerosol mask
6-8. Tachycardia, for an adult, is defined as a heart rate greater than which of the following minimal values?
  A. 60 beats/min
  B. 80 beats/min
  C. 100 beats/min
  D. 120 beats/min
6-9. Tachycardia is least likely to result from which of the following?
  A. hypothermia
  B. hypoxemia
  C. exercise
  D. fear
6-10. Bradypnea is least likely to occur in patients with which of the following?
  A. head injury
  B. metabolic acidosis
  C. hypothermia
  D. drug overdose

6-11. Pulsus paradoxus may occur in all of the following except:
   A. chronic obstructive pulmonary disease or asthma
   B. cardiac tamponade
   C. peripheral vascular disease
   D. constrictive pericarditis

6-12. Scoliosis refers to which of the following?
   A. a funnel-shaped depression on the sternum
   B. a lateral curvature of the spine
   C. a forward projection of the sternum
   D. an A-P curvature of the spine

6-13. Yellow sputum indicates which of the following?
   A. normal sputum color
   B. old retained secretions
   C. an acute infection
   D. old blood

6-14. Which of the following would not be an indication of respiratory distress?
   A. use of accessory muscles
   B. pursed lip breathing
   C. chest retractions
   D. presence of vesicular breath sounds

6-15. During palpation, it is noted that a patient's trachea is deviated to the right. This may be caused by which of the following?
   A. a tension pneumothorax on the right
   B. a tumor mass on the right
   C. pleural effusion on the right
   D. atelectasis on the right

6-16. Which of the following would tend to increase tactile fremitus?
   A. alveolar consolidation
   B. thick pleural lining
   C. pneumothorax
   D. obese chest wall

6-17. A patient suffering from a pneumothorax would have which type of percussion note?
   A. flat
   B. short
   C. hyperresonant
   D. high pitched

6-18. More than 80% of all bacterial pneumonias are caused by which of the following?
   A. *Legionella pneumophila*
   B. *Pseudomonas aeruginosa*
   C. Staphylococcus
   D. Streptococcus

6-19. Milky pleural fluid is associated with which of the following?
   A. heart failure
   B. liver disease
   C. lymph flow (chyle) leakage
   D. pulmonary infarction

6-20. A transudate, in the pleural cavity, would most likely be caused by which of the following?
   A. infection
   B. congestive heart failure (CHF)
   C. cancer
   D. trauma

Match the Following:

Breath Sounds

_____ 6-21. Crackles

_____ 6-22. Diminished

_____ 6-23. Wheeze

_____ 6-24. Bronchial

_____ 6-25. Pleural friction rub

_____ 6-26. Rhonchi

_____ 6-27. Vesicular

_____ 6-28. Adventitious

Definitions

A. normal over trachea, abnormal over lung periphery

B. general term used to describe abnormal breath sounds

C. decreased breath sounds

D. caused by air entering previously closed alveoli, often associated with "wet" lungs

E. term used to describe normal peripheral breath sounds

F. high-pitched sounds caused by narrowed airways with gas flow at a high velocity

G. sound similar to leather being rubbed together

H. low-pitched sounds often caused by air flowing over secretions may be cleared with coughing

DOCUMENTATION: CASE STUDY 1

S: "About an hour ago, while I was carrying a bag of groceries, I got this sharp pain in my right chest and at the same time, I got short of breath."

O: 35-year-old slender white woman in moderate respiratory distress. Monitor reveals sinus tachycardia. All other vital signs within normal limits. Examination reveals respiratory movement is greater in right chest and tracheal deviation to the left. Breath sounds normal over left lung fields and diminished in the right upper lobe. Chest radiograph reveals a partial pneumothorax in right upper lobe.

A: Partial pneumothorax in right upper lobe; moderate respiratory distress.

P:
1. Administer O_2 at 2 L/min.
2. Collaborate with health care team to insert chest tube
3. Admit

DOCUMENTATION: CASE STUDY 2

S: "I'm having trouble breathing."

O: The patient is a poorly nourished, unkempt white man who appears older than his stated age. Patient is alert, oriented, and in severe respiratory distress during the physical examination. Monitor reveals sinus tachycardia at 126/minute, temperature is 38.7°C, respirations 28/min, and blood pressure 154/96. Examination reveals anterior diameter of chest is equal to posterior diameter. Chest expansion is symmetrical. Normal resonance to percussion over most of the chest except the right lower chest which has decreased resonance. Breath sounds diminished with scattered high-pitched wheezes throughout all lung fields. Fine crackles in right lower lobe. Course rhonchi and bronchial breath sounds in left lower lobe. There is nail-bed cyanosis of fingers. No clubbing. +1 pitting edema of ankles. Pulses are +2 in all areas except for dorsalis pedis pulses, which are +1. Chest radiograph shows changes consistent with emphysema. There is consolidation of right lower lobe consistent with lobar pneumonia.

A: Emphysema with right lobar pneumonia; moderate respiratory distress.

P:
1. Obtain ABG
2. Administer O_2 at 2 L/min; consult with physician and adjust as needed as per ABG
3. Collaborate with health care team in the administration of bronchodilators, antibiotics, diuretics, and digoxin
4. Admit

7

Imaging Assessment

BASIC PRINCIPLES

The chest radiograph is the most common imaging technique used for looking at structures inside the chest. X-rays are radiant energy consisting of wavelengths shorter than ultraviolet light. Because of their short wavelength, x-rays will penetrate many substances. The x-ray energy that penetrates an object is recorded on a special photographic film that is held inside a cassette or plate. A film that is unexposed (no x-rays have reached it) is white. A film that is completely exposed turns black. When a radiograph is taken, substances that block most x-ray penetration (radiopaque) will appear white on the film. Substances that allow x-rays to pass through them (radiolucent) will appear black. Object density and thickness are the two main factors affecting the amount of x-ray penetration that will occur. As density or thickness increases, penetration will decrease and the film will appear white. Differentiation of structures within the chest can made because of their varied density or thickness. This is known as *contrast.* The *silhouette sign* is the loss of distinct appearance of a common border. Normally the heart and lungs have a distinct border owing to difference in density. If the heart border cannot be seen on the right or left (silhouette sign), the infiltrate is in the right middle lobe or the left Lingula, respectively. If a pulmonary infiltrate is posterior to the heart, the heart border should be visible.

POSITIONING FOR RADIOGRAPH

A common position for an outpatient chest radiograph is the PA (posteroanterior) exposure. With this technique, the patient stands with his or her chest against the cassette and the x-ray beam passes through the patient's back to their front (posterior to anterior) and then onto the film. The AP (anteroposterior) chest film is much more common in the intensive care unit. Here, the cassette is placed behind the patient and the beam is directed toward the patient's front. The PA exposure is taken from a distance of 6 feet. The AP is taken from a distance of 4 feet. The closer an object is to the film, the smaller and sharper it will appear. This is important since the heart sits more toward the anterior chest wall. An AP film will show the heart as slightly larger than on a PA film. Be careful not to interpret an enlarged heart on the AP film just because of the technique used.

The lateral radiograph is taken from a side view of the patient. A left lateral is commonly performed, which means that the patient's left side is on the plate and the beam enters from the right side. The oblique technique is a PA exposure, but the patient is turned a quarter turn, which lifts one side of the thorax off the plate. The lateral decubitus technique has the patient lying down on his or her side for the exposure. The beam is directed in a PA fashion. Lordotic films are an AP exposure, but instead of the beam being projected in a horizontal direction (90° angle), it is projected at an upward angle (120° angle) in relation to the chest.

VIEWING FILMS

When looking at x-ray films, AP and PA films are always viewed as if the patient is facing you. Lateral films can be viewed as if the patient is looking in either direction. Magnetic resonance imaging (MRI) and computed tomography (CT) scan films are viewed as though the patient is lying down on his or her back and you are looking from a caudal to cephalic view. (A cross-sectional view, observing from the patient's feet up toward his or her head.)

NORMAL RADIOGRAPHIC FEATURES

When interpreting chest radiographs, the normal structures must be known so that abnormalities can be distinguished.

1. The right diaphragm is higher than the left (by 2 cm).
2. The costophrenic angles should be clear (it takes approximately 200 mL of fluid to blunt the angles).

3. The left hilum is higher than the right (by 2 cm).
4. The trachea is midline and filled with air.
5. The aortic arch is left of the spine.
6. The heart lies more toward the left thorax.
7. There is often a gastric air bubble on the left side of the abdomen.
8. Paired structures should look like each other.

LUNG FISSURES

There is one main fissure in the left lung. It is the major or oblique fissure separating the upper lobe and ligula from the lower lobe. In the right lung, there are two main fissures. The major or oblique fissure separates the upper and middle lobes from the lower lobe. The minor or horizontal fissure separates the right upper lobe from the right middle lobe. These fissures may be seen on a normal radiograph but become more prominent when thickened, filled with fluid, or consolidation is present.

REVIEW QUESTIONS

7-1. Which of the following would have the greatest radio-opacity?
   A. body fluids
   B. fatty tissue
   C. barium
   D. calcium
7-2. The chest radiographs of patients with the following diseases may all appear normal except:
   A. severe emphysema
   B. severe chronic bronchitis
   C. severe asthma
   D. early lung carcinoma
7-3. An AP chest film will differ from a PA film in all of the following except that the AP film will not have:
   A. high clavicles
   B. the scapulae overlying lung fields
   C. diaphragmatic elevation
   D. a smaller heart shadow
7-4. Which of the following may better demonstrate small pleural effusion presence?
   A. oblique projection
   B. lordotic projection
   C. lateral decubitus view
   D. end-expiratory film
7-5. Which of the following may aid in detection of a small pneumothorax?
   A. oblique projection
   B. lordotic projection
   C. lateral decubitus view
   D. end-expiratory film

7-6. The gold standard for detection of deep vein thrombosis is:
   A. bronchography
   B. pulmonary arteriography
   C. venography
   D. bronchial arteriography
7-7. The noninvasive technique of choice for detection of deep vein thrombosis (DVT) is which of the following?
   A. doppler ultrasonography
   B. CT scan
   C. MRI
   D. fluoroscopy
7-8. Which of the following opacifications would most likely result in "loss of volume" as interpreted from an x-ray film?
   A. consolidation
   B. replacement opacity
   C. pleural effusion
   D. atelectasis
7-9. The direct roentgenographic sign of atelectasis is which of the following?
   A. hilar shift
   B. contralateral lung hyperinflation
   C. decrease in size of a rib interspace
   D. increased opacification
7-10. Indirect roentgenographic signs of atelectasis include each of the following except:
   A. elevation of the hemidiaphragm on the affected side
   B. shift of the mediastinum away from the affected side
   C. hyperinflation of adjacent lobes
   D. a shift of the hilum
7-11. Hyperinflation of the lung manifests itself on radiograph by each of the following except:
   A. flattening of the diaphragm
   B. increased translucency of the lung fields
   C. increased vascular markings
   D. increased retrosternal air space
7-12. An exudative effusion may be caused by each of the following except:
   A. pneumonia
   B. mycobacterial infections
   C. pleural mesothelioma
   D. left heart failure
7-13. Bilateral elevation of the diaphragm would likely be caused by each of the following except:
   A. severe asthma
   B. pulmonary embolism
   C. obesity
   D. ascites
7-14. A tension pneumothorax would result in which of the following?
   A. absence of lung markings on the affected side
   B. mediastinal shift toward the unaffected side
   C. flattened diaphragm on the affected side
   D. all of the above

8

Pulmonary Function Tests

Pulmonary function tests (PFTs) are an intricate part of overall patient assessment. Although some think PFT is a specialty area of respiratory care, having knowledge of PFTs and being able to interpret them is important for all respiratory care practitioners (RCPs) who are involved in patient care. PFTs are not routinely done to diagnose a problem, but to test the severity of a suspected disease or condition based on patient history and assessment. Some reasons for performing PFTs would include the following: determination of presence of pulmonary disease, following the course of a disease, checking response to medication, a pre/postsurgical evaluation, and disability evaluation.

LUNG VOLUMES AND CAPACITIES

Each lung volume and capacity has a definition explaining what each represents. I would suggest that students memorize each of these definitions. Actual values for these parameters will vary from individual to individual depending on actual lung size, which is influenced mostly by age, height, gender, and ethnic background. Lung volume values are proportional to height, and inversely proportional to age after age 20 to 25 years. (I often tell my students they are already over the hill and they don't even know it.) Males, keeping other factors the same, have larger lung volumes than females. Individuals with some ethnic backgrounds (black, Asian, and East Indies) routinely have smaller lung volumes, and a correction factor should be used if white (caucasian) predicted values are used. Volume nomograms for children are often based on height alone.

Lung volumes can be measured directly or indirectly. Direct measurements are values that can be measured directly from a spirogram tracing. Indirect measurements cannot be measured from a spirogram but are measured using other means such as helium dilution, nitrogen washout, or a body box. Lung volumes are referenced from the "base line" or resting level of breathing at end exhalation. This resting level of breathing is determined when the outward expansion force of the chest wall is balanced by the inward recoil force of the lungs, while the respiratory muscles are at rest.

Lung volumes

See Figure 8-1.

Tidal volume (VT): The volume of air (gas) normally inhaled from the resting level of breathing. (Of course, the exhaled value, back to base line, would also be called VT.)

Inspiratory reserve volume (IRV): The maximum volume of air that can be inhaled following an inhaled VT.

Expiratory reserve volume (ERV): The maximum volume of air that can be exhaled from the resting level of breathing.

Residual volume (RV): The volume of air remaining in the lungs after a maximal exhalation. (After the ERV maneuver.)

Lung Capacities

See Figure 8-1.

Each capacity is made up of two or more lung volumes or a combination of volumes and capacities.

Inspiratory capacity (IC): The maximum amount of air that can be inhaled from the resting level of breathing.

Functional residual capacity (FRC): The volume of air remaining in the lungs at the resting level of breathing.

Vital capacity (VC): The maximum amount of air that can be exhaled following a maximum inspiration. It can also be defined as the maximum amount of air that can be inhaled following a maximum exhalation.

Total lung capacity (TLC): The amount of air in the lungs following a maximum inspiration.

Once the lung volumes and capacities are realized the following formulas can be used. These are only examples of many possible combinations.

$$VT + IRV = IC \text{ and } TLC - FRC = IC$$

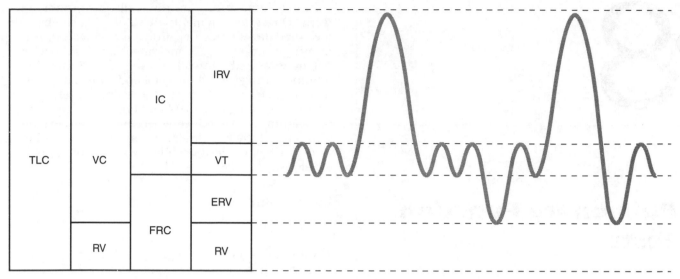

FIGURE 8-1. Lung volumes and capacities illustrated as a bar graph and as a spirogram.

$$RV + ERV = FRC \text{ and } TLC - IC = FRC$$

$$IRV + V_T + ERV = VC \text{ and } IC + ERV = VC \text{ and}$$
$$TLC - RV = VC$$

$$IRV + V_T + ERV + RV = TLC$$

Considering the previous parameters, the following are direct measurements and can be measured from a spirogram tracing: IRV, V_T, ERV, IC, and VC.

Because RV cannot be exhaled, it cannot be measured from a spirogram. Therefore, the following are classified as indirect measurements: RV, FRC, and TLC.

Vital Capacity: Volume-Time Tracing

VC has already been defined. It is routinely measured as an expiratory maneuver. It can be performed as a slow or rapid (forced) maneuver. Just as a rose by any other name is still a rose, a VC, whether slow (SVC) or forced (FVC), inspiratory (IVC), or expiratory (EVC), is still a VC. There are reasons for doing both slow and forced maneuvers. A patient with obstructive lung disease will often be able to exhale more air while performing a SVC than an FVC. This is because a forced maneuver results in dynamic airway collapse, trapping air in the lungs and decreasing the volume of exhaled air. It is important when performing an FVC to give as much effort as possible and to continue to exhale until empty.

Forced expiratory volume in 1 second (FEV_1) is the volume of air exhaled in the first second of the FVC maneuver. The FEV_1 should be thought of as a volume measurement, but since it is a volume/time parameter it can also be considered as the average flow during the first second of exhalation. FEV_2 is the volume exhaled in 2 seconds, and FEV_3 is the volume exhaled in 3 seconds.

Forced expiratory flow 25–75 (FEF_{25-75}) is the average flow rate in L/sec during the mid 50% of the FVC. To manually measure this value, you need to locate the middle 50% of the FVC volume, then determine the time it took to exhale that volume. FEF_{25-75} equals mid 50% of volume (L)/time (sec).

Forced expiratory time (FET) is the total time spent in the expiratory phase.

Except for the VC, each of the previous values can only be measured from the volume-time tracing.

Vital Capacity: Flow-Volume Tracing

Except for the VC, each of the following can only be measured from the flow-volume curve.

Peak expiratory flow (PEF) is the measurement of the highest flow rate achieved during exhalation and is very effort dependent. The greater the patient effort, the higher the flow.

Forced expiratory flow 25 (FEF_{25}) is the flow rate measured after having exhaled 25% of the FVC.

Forced expiratory flow 50 (FEF_{50}) is the flow rate measured after having exhaled 50% of the FVC.

Forced expiratory flow 75 (FEF_{75}) is the flow rate measured after having exhaled 75% of the FVC.

Please check the text of *Respiratory Care* for measuring procedures. You will have the opportunity to practice measurement of these parameters later in this chapter.

TABLE 8-1 **A Guide for PFT Interpretation**

Parameter	Obstruction	Restriction	Mixed
VC	N/D	D	D
FEV_1	D	D	D
FEV_1:FVC	D	N/I	D
RV,FRC	I	D	D
Flows	D	N/D	D

Where: D = decreased; I = increased; N = normal

PFT INTERPRETATION

Interpretation of PFTs can be involved, but it can also be simplified by considering a few basic elements. In general, obstructive defects have a VC that is normal or decreased, an RV or FRC that is normal or increased, an FEV_1:FVC ratio that is decreased, and flow rates that are decreased. Restrictive defects have volumes that are decreased, an FEV_1:FVC ratio that is normal, and flow rates that are normal or decreased. (Flow rates can be decreased as the restriction progresses to moderate and severe. There is just not enough volume present to generate normal flows.) Mixed defects have decreased volumes, a decreased FEV_1:FVC ratio, and decreased flows. This is of course an oversimplification but will go a long way in helping to interpret PFTs. Refer to Table 8-1 for a summary of PFT results for lung disease.

FRC DETERMINATION

Helium dilution is probably the most common method used to determine FRC. Helium is a good gas to use for the test for three basic reasons. First, its decreased density may help in its distribution in the lung, thus giving a truer indication of the size of the FRC. Second, it is inert, which means little helium will dissolve in the blood stream or other tissue. If large amounts of helium left the lung and dissolved in the body tissue, it would be difficult to know how much helium was actually diluted in the lungs' FRC. A large correction factor would be needed to try to estimate the FRC. Third, it is also nontoxic, but do not try to breathe 100% helium without oxygen present.

DIFFUSION CAPACITY

Diffusion of a gas is addressed by Ficks' Law.

$$D \propto (SA \times \Delta P)/T$$

where:

D is the diffusion of a gas in mL/min/mmHg

SA is the surface area where $\dot{V}/\dot{Q}$ matching allows diffusion to occur

ΔP is the pressure difference between the alveolar gas partial pressure and plasma gas partial pressure

T is the thickness of the A-C membrane

A common method used to measure diffusion rate in the lungs is the single breath carbon monoxide diffusion test (DLCOSB). This test uses a gas mixture of approximately 10% helium, 0.3% CO, 21% oxygen, and the balance is nitrogen. The test involves exhaling to RV, rapidly inhaling the gas mixture to TLC, maintaining a breath hold for 10 seconds, and exhaling again, rapidly. Part of the exhaled gas is captured for analysis. CO is a good gas to use in this test for several reasons. First, except for a small amount, CO is a nonresident gas in the lung and body. This makes it easy to track and measure without the need for correction factors. Second, CO has a diffusion rate similar to oxygen (the gas which we are really interested in knowing the diffusion rate of). Actually, oxygen diffuses 1.23 times faster than CO. Third, CO has a great affinity for hemoglobin. CO has 210 times the affinity for hemoglobin compared with oxygen. This means it will bind with hemoglobin much more readily and does not want to break its attachment. Finally, CO is a diffusion-limited gas. This means that the only factor that limits the amount of CO that will enter the blood stream is ability to diffuse. This is in contrast to oxygen, which is a perfusion-limited gas. The amount of oxygen that is able to enter the blood stream is dependent not only on its ability to diffuse but on the perfusion of the blood as well. When oxygen enters the blood stream, it builds up a partial pressure (back pressure) in the plasma. When the partial pressure of oxygen in the plasma equals the alveolar partial pressure of oxygen (zero diffusion gradient), diffusion stops. This does not happen with CO. Because of the low percentage of CO used in the test, the short time of the test, and the great affinity of hemoglobin for CO, virtually all the CO that crosses the A-C membrane attaches to hemoglobin, thus keeping the plasma partial pressure of CO near zero. This allows CO to continue to diffuse as long as blood is in contact with the alveolar space.

The other gas that is part of the gas mixture in the diffusion test, which may raise questions as to why it is used, is helium. The properties of helium were discussed previously. One of those properties was that it is inert. This is important for the diffusion test. When helium is inhaled, it is diluted by the patient's RV. If 10% helium is inhaled, only 7% helium will be exhaled because it was diluted by the patient's RV. (The actual percentage of helium exhaled will vary depending on the size of the RV and VC). You can actually calculate the size of the patient's RV from the measurements of the inhaled and exhaled helium concentrations. This process may underestimate the actual RV size, especially in patients with obstructive airway disease. When CO is inhaled, it is also diluted by the patient's RV, but CO also diffuses across the A-C membrane. When a patient inhales 0.3% CO and exhales 0.1% CO, it is reduced for two reasons, dilution and diffusion. How much of the decrease is caused by dilution and how much is caused by diffusion? The helium allows us to calculate how much of the decrease in CO is caused by dilution. The rest of the decrease of CO is caused by diffusion. In reality, the calculation of the DLCOSB is an indirect measurement based on the helium dilution.

There are numerous factors that will decrease the diffusion capacity. A few are mentioned here. Patients with anemia (decreased red blood cells or hemoglobin) will have a decreased diffusion capacity. With less hemoglobin available, there are fewer sites for CO to bind to hemoglobin. This results in more of the CO remaining in the plasma, causing an increase in back pressure. In this situation, CO starts to behave more like a perfusion-limited gas, and diffusion rates drop. Individuals who smoke have a similar problem because they have a chronically elevated CO level, and many hemoglobin sites are already bound by CO. Patients who smoke should refrain from smoking for at least 24 hours before the test. If an arterial blood gas test is done at the time of testing, a correction factor can be used to adjust the measured values, much like it can be done for anemia. Some other causes of a decreased diffusion rate include the following: a thickened A-C membrane (interstitial lung disease), loss of lung volume (pneumonectomy, atelectasis), loss of A-C membrane (emphysema), and increased $\dot{V}/\dot{Q}$ mismatch (pulmonary emboli).

To help determine if a decreased DLCO is only caused by the loss of lung volume or if it is because of other reasons, the diffusion rate:lung volume (DL:VA) ratio can be calculated. (DL is the diffusion rate and VA is the alveolar volume—TLC at standard temperature and pressure, dry (STPD)—at which the DLCO was measured.) If the DLCO is decreased owing to loss of lung volume only, the DL:VA will be normal. If, on the other hand, the DLCO is decreased because of factors other than loss of lung volume, the DL:VA will be decreased as well.

Example

Patient A has a predicted DLCO of 26 mL/min/mmHg and an actual of 14, which is 54% of normal. The predicted DL:VA is 5.2 and the actual is 2.3 (44%).

Patient B has a predicted DLCO 20 mL/min/mmHg and an actual of 12, which is 60% of normal. The predicted DL:VA for patient B is 4.5 and his actual was 4.0 (89%). Patient B has a decreased DLCO owing to loss of lung volume, whereas patient A has a decreased DLCO for reasons other than just loss of lung volume.

STPD, ATPS, AND BTPS

STPD is standard temperature and pressure, dry
    Standard temperature is 0°C
    Standard pressure is one atmospheric pressure at 760 mmHg
    Dry means there is no water vapor ($PH_2O = 0$)
ATPS is ambient temperature, pressure, saturated
    Ambient temperature is the temperature for the given situation
    Ambient pressure is the actual pressure of the given situation
    Saturated means that the gas at the given temperature is carrying all the water it can (RH = 100%)
BTPS is body temperature, pressure, saturated
    Body temperature is routinely 37°C
    Body pressure is ambient pressure
    Saturated means that the gas at 37°C is carrying all the water that it can
    (RH = 100%)

PF volume-collecting devices collect exhaled gas samples at near ATPS (room) conditions, but all PFT values are reported at BTPS (except the DLCO and the DL:VA, which historically have been reported at STPD). BTPS values are larger than ATPS values because a volume of gas expands as it is heated and as moisture is added (Charles' Law). This means that a correction factor must be used. Most PFT equipment is now computerized, and the correction to BTPS is done automatically and correctly as long as the appropriate factors are used. If performing the calculation manually, the following chart lists a few correction factors based on the ambient temperature. The given correction factors need to be multiplied with the ATPS volume measurements to equal the BTPS volume values (Table 8-2).

TABLE 8-2 **ATPS to BTPS Volume Conversion Factors for Common Ambient Temperatures at or near 760 mmHg Pressure**

Temperature (°C)	BTPS Factor
20	1.102
21	1.096
22	1.091
23	1.085
24	1.080
25	1.075
26	1.068

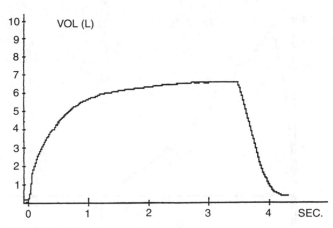

FIGURE 8-2. Volume–time curve.

CALCULATION EXERCISES

Lung Volume and Capacity Calculations

Given the following, determine the lung volumes and capacities listed.

	Given	**Determine**
8-1.	VC = 4.18 L	$V_T \approx$ ___ L
	IRV = 2.62 L	RV $\approx$ ___ L
	TLC = 5.12 L	FRC $\approx$ ___ L
	ERV = 1.05 L	IC $\approx$ ___ L
8-2.	TLC = 5.77 L	RV $\approx$ ___ L
	VC = 4.60 L	ERV $\approx$ ___ L
	FRC = 2.37 L	IC $\approx$ ___ L
	IRV = 2.87 L	$V_T \approx$ ___ L
8-3.	FRC = 2.86 L	RV $\approx$ ___ L
	ERV = 1.46 L	VC $\approx$ ___ L
	V_T = 0.30 L	IC $\approx$ ___ L
	IRV = 3.16 L	TLC $\approx$ ___ L
8-4.	VC = 4.48 L	TLC $\approx$ ___ L
	RV = 1.14 L	ERV $\approx$ ___ L
	FRC = 2.21 L	IRV $\approx$ ___ L
	V_T = 0.57 L	IC $\approx$ ___ L
8-5.	V_T = 0.47 L	IC $\approx$ ___ L
	IRV = 3.00 L	VC $\approx$ ___ L
	ERV = 0.99 L	FRC $\approx$ ___ L
	RV = 1.01 L	TLC $\approx$ ___ L
8-6.	TLC = 6.30 L	RV $\approx$ ___ L
	VC = 5.18 L	ERV $\approx$ ___ L
	FRC = 2.54 L	IC $\approx$ ___ L
	IRV = 3.29 L	$V_T \approx$ ___ L
8-7.	VC = 4.38 L	TLC $\approx$ ___ L
	RV = 1.04 L	ERV $\approx$ ___ L
	FRC = 1.96 L	IRV $\approx$ ___ L
	V_T = 0.39 L	IC $\approx$ ___ L

Volume–Time Curve Calculations

From the following volume–time curve (Figure 8–2) determine each of the parameters listed below.

8-8. FVC $\approx$ ___ L

8-9. $FEV_1 \approx$ ___ L

8-10. $FEV_1 / FVC \approx$ ___ %

8-11. $FEV_2 \approx$ ___ L

8-12. $FEV_3 \approx$ ___ L

8-13. $FEF_{25-75} \approx$ ___ L/sec

8-14. FET $\approx$ ___ sec

Flow–Volume Curve Calculations

From the following flow–volume curve (Figure 8-3) determine each of the parameters listed below.

8-15. FVC $\approx$ ___ L

8-16. PEF $\approx$ ___ L/sec

8-17. $FEF_{25} \approx$ ___ L/sec

8-18. $FEF_{50} \approx$ ___ L/sec

8-19. $FEF_{75} \approx$ ___ L/sec

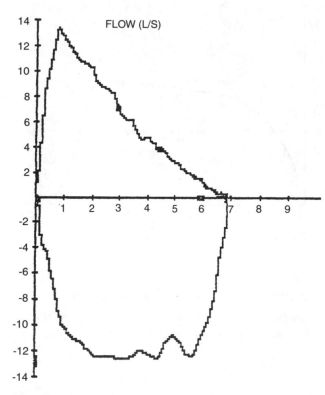

FIGURE 8-3. Flow–volume curve.

PFT Interpretations

Interpret each of the following as normal, restricted, obstructed, or mixed.

	Parameter	Actual	Pre-dicted	% Pre-dicted
8-20.	SVC	5.74 L	5.12 L	112
	FVC	5.79 L	5.12 L	113
	FEV$_1$	5.17 L	4.46 L	116
	FEV$_1$:FVC	89%	87%	—
	FEF$_{25-75}$	5.87 L/sec	5.46 L/sec	108
	Interpretation:			
8-21.	SVC	2.90 L	3.64 L	80
	FVC	2.43 L	3.64 L	67
	FEV$_1$	0.38 L	2.86 L	13
	FEV$_1$:FVC	16%	79%	—
	FEF$_{25-75}$	0.11 L/sec	3.83 L/sec	3
	Interpretation:			
8-22.	SVC	2.45 L	3.64 L	67
	FVC	2.37 L	3.64 L	65
	FEV$_1$	1.97 L	2.80 L	70
	FEV$_1$:FVC	83%	77%	—
	FEF$_{25-75}$	2.99 L/sec	3.65 L/sec	82
	Interpretation:			
8-23.	SVC	1.50 L	2.46 L	61
	FVC	1.50 L	2.46 L	61
	FEV$_1$	1.02 L	1.90 L	54
	FEV$_1$:FVC	68%	77%	—
	FEF$_{25-75}$	0.62 L/sec	2.65 L/sec	23
	Interpretation:			
8-24.	SVC	2.27 L	2.46 L	92
	FVC	2.36 L	2.46 L	96
	FEV$_1$	1.86 L	1.96 L	94
	FEV$_1$:FVC	78%	79%	—
	FEF$_{25-75}$	1.71 L/sec	2.78 L/sec	62
	Interpretation:			

Lung Volume and Capacity Determinations

Determine the following:

8-25. IC + ERV = ___

8-26. FRC – RV = ___

8-27. FRC + IC = ___

8-28. TLC – IC = ___

8-29. IRV + V$_T$ + FRC = ___

8-30. VC – IC = ___

8-31. IC – V$_T$ = ___

8-32. TLC – VC = ___

REVIEW QUESTIONS

8-33. Which of the following is not correct concerning the diffusion of CO?
   A. D$_L$CO is increased in emphysema
   B. D$_L$CO is normal in simple bronchitis
   C. D$_L$CO is normal or increased in asthma
   D. D$_L$CO is decreased in interstitial lung disease

8-34. Which of the following is not a major factor in determining lung volumes?
   A. height
   B. weight
   C. age
   D. gender

8-35. The volume of air remaining in the lungs after a maximal exhalation is:
   A. V$_T$
   B. ERV
   C. RV
   D. FRC

8-36. TLC is equal to:
- A. VC − RV
- B. IC + FRC
- C. IRV + V_T + ERV
- D. V_T + FRC

8-37. Which of the following is not an indirect measurement?
- A. TLC
- B. RV
- C. FRC
- D. IC

8-38. Which of the following is incorrect?
- A. PF tests may determine presence of pulmonary disease before the onset of signs and symptoms
- B. lung function may improve if an individual stops smoking
- C. PF tests may help identify patients at risk for surgery
- D. PF tests cannot help differentiate between cardiac and pulmonary causes of shortness of breath (SOB)

8-39. Considering the FVC, which of the following is incorrect?
- A. the maneuver requires considerable patient cooperation
- B. there must be at least three acceptable maneuvers
- C. there must be three reproducible maneuvers
- D. if unacceptable results after eight attempts patient should be rescheduled

8-40. Which of the following is not correct?
- A. PEF is an effort independent parameter
- B. a decreased FEF_{25-75} is often caused by airway obstruction
- C. an increased FEV_1:FVC ratio can be observed in restrictive defects
- D. FET may take 20 seconds in severe obstruction

8-41. Which of the following is not correct concerning the forced inspiratory vital capacity (FIVC)?
- A. it is indicated whenever an upper airway obstruction is suspected
- B. the maneuver is very effort dependent
- C. it should be used for general screening of outpatients
- D. the shape of the FIVC curve is the most important aspect of the maneuver

8-42. Which of the following is not correct concerning the maximal inspiratory pressure (MIP) and maximal expiratory pressure (MEP) maneuvers?
- A. they are indicated when respiratory muscle weakness is suspected
- B. the MIP maneuver starts at the level of the FRC
- C. the MEP maneuver starts at the level of the TLC
- D. decreased values may be due to decreased respiratory muscle strength

8-43. Diffusion of a gas is inversely proportional to which of the following?
- A. surface area
- B. pressure gradient
- C. thickness of the membrane
- D. solubility coefficient

8-44. A volume of 5.0 L at ATPS (temperature 24°C) will be what volume when corrected to BTPS?
- A. 5.4 L
- B. 5.2 L
- C. 5.0 L
- D. 4.7 L

9

Arterial Blood Gas Analysis

PARTIAL PRESSURE, FRACTIONAL, AND PERCENT CONCENTRATIONS OF GAS CALCULATIONS AND EXERCISES

Determination of the Partial Pressure of a Gas (Pgas)

Room air contains approximately 21% O_2 (FO_2 = 0.21) and 79% N_2 (FN_2 = 0.79). To determine the partial pressure exerted by a gas, when the fractional concentration is known, use the following formula:

$$Pt \times Fgas = Pgas$$

where:

Pt is the total pressure of a system, in this case, atmospheric pressure (Patm)

Fgas is the fractional concentration of a gas, and

Pgas is the partial pressure of a gas based on its fractional concentration

Example

Given Patm = 760 mmHg, FO_2 = 0.21 and FN_2 = 0.79

760 mmHg × 0.21 = 160 mmHg (PO_2), and

760 mmHg × 0.79 = 600 mmHg (PN_2)

This partial pressure of oxygen is actually the pressure of inspired oxygen and is designated as PiO_2. The PN_2 is the pressure of inspired nitrogen and is designated as PiN_2.

Determination of the Fractional Concentration of a Gas (Fgas)

The Fgas can be determined if the Pt and Pgas are known by using the following formula:

$$Pgas/Pt = Fgas$$

Example

Given PO_2 = 160 mmHg and Pt = 760 mmHg, calculate FO_2.

160 mmHg (PO_2)/760 mmHg (Pt) = 0.21 (FO_2) or 21% O_2

(Where Fgas × 100 = % gas)

Partial Pressure and Percent Calculations

9-1. Calculate the partial pressure of O_2 (PO_2) and N_2 (PN_2) in a 50%/50% O_2/N_2 mixture, where the total pressure (Pt) is 740 mmHg._____

_____

_____

_____

9-2. Calculate the PHe and PO_2 in a 70%/30% He/O_2 gas mixture, where the Pt is 780 mmHg.

_____

_____

_____

9-3. Calculate Pt, FO_2, $\%O_2$, FCO_2, $\%CO_2$, FN_2, and $\%N_2$, if PO_2 is 70 mmHg, PCO_2 is 30 mmHg, and PN_2 is 520 mmHg. _____

_____

_____

_____

9-4. If 100% O_2 is being delivered to a patient and the Pt is 760, what is the PO_2? _____

_____

_____

_____

Calculation of Pt is an application of Dalton's Law that states that the total system pressure is equal to the sum of all the partial pressures of the gases present.

ALVEOLAR AIR EQUATION

The partial pressure of oxygen in the environment (PIO_2) will have a direct effect on the partial pressure of oxygen in the alveoli (PAO_2). The PAO_2 will then have a direct effect on the arterial oxygen tension (PaO_2). We know from our former discussion that $Patm \times FIO_2 = PIO_2$. This describes the partial pressure of O_2 in the inspired gas under dry conditions. This formula must now be modified to include water vapor. For normal patient situations, water vapor pressure (PH_2O) is 47 mmHg at 37°C and 100% relative humidity. The modified formula will now appear like this:

$$(Patm - 47) \times FIO_2 = PIO_2$$

This calculation reduces the PIO_2 of air (dry) from 160 mmHg ($760 \times 0.21 = 160$), to a PIO_2 of air (humidified) of 150 mmHg ($[760 - 47] \times 0.21 = 150$).

The alveolar air equation takes the above formula one step further and allows the calculation of PAO_2 (the partial pressure of oxygen in the alveoli). It is based on the Patm, FIO_2, $PaCO_2$, and the R factor and is expressed in the following formula:

$$PAO_2 = (Patm - 47)(FIO_2) - PaCO_2$$
$$(FIO_2 + [(1 - FIO_2)/R])$$

This formula is often simplified to the following form:

$$PAO_2 = (Patm - 47)(FIO_2) - PaCO_2/R$$

Where:

PAO_2 is the alveolar PO_2 in mmHg

Patm is atmospheric pressure or the barometric pressure (pressure measured by a barometer), expressed in mmHg. In this case, it is also the absolute pressure to which the patient is exposed.

47 is the water vapor pressure (PH_2O) in mmHg in a person's lungs at 37°C and 100% relative humidity (RII)

FIO_2 is the fractional concentration of inhaled O_2

$PaCO_2$ is the arterial CO_2 value in mmHg

R is the respiratory exchange ratio (RER) the actual mean ratio of CO_2/O_2 exchanged in the lung.

Note: There are several factors that will affect the actual R value, and discussion of them is beyond the scope of this text. 0.8 is considered normal and is commonly used in the formula unless the patients actual R value is known. When patients are breathing 100% O_2, R will be given a value of one (1), thus eliminating it from the formula.

Examples

Example A
While breathing room air at 1 Patm of 760 mmHg, the PIO_2 is approximately 150 mmHg. A person with a normal $PaCO_2$ of 40 mmHg will have a PAO_2 of approximately 100 mmHg.

$$PAO_2 = (760 - 47)(0.21) - 40/0.8$$
$$PAO_2 = 713 \times 0.21 - 50$$
$$PAO_2 = 150 - 50 = 100 \text{ mmHg}$$

Example B

Breathing room air (21% O_2) at 1 Patm of 640 mmHg and having a $PaCO_2$ of 40 results in the following values: PIO_2 of 125 and a PAO_2 of 75.

$PAO_2 = (640 - 47)(0.21) - 40/0.8$

$PAO_2 = 593 \times 0.21 - 50$

$PAO_2 = 125 - 50 = 75$ mmHg

Note that PH_2O does not change with changes in pressure.

Example C

Breathing 100% O_2 at 760 mmHg with a $PaCO_2$ of 60 mmHg.

$PAO_2 = (760 - 47)(1.0) - 60$

$PAO_2 = 713 \times 1 - 60$

$PAO_2 = 713 - 60 = 653$ mmHg

Remember that R = 1 for this calculation.

PIO_2 and PAO_2 Calculations

Calculate the PIO_2 and PAO_2 for each of the following conditions. PH_2O will be 47 mmHg for each of the calculations.

	Patm (mmHg)	FIO_2	$PaCO_2$ (mmHg)	PIO_2 (mmHg)	PAO_2 (mmHg)
9-5.	760	.30	40	____	____
9-6.	760	1.0	40	____	____
9-7.	760	.30	80	____	____
9-8.	640	.21	60	____	____
9-9.	640	.50	40	____	____
9-10.	620	.21	20	____	____
9-11.	760	.21	20	____	____
9-12.	760	.70	40	____	____

a/A RATIO AND A-a GRADIENT

PAO_2 will have a direct effect on PaO_2. Two of several methods used to assess how well the lungs are able to oxygenate the blood involve the measurement of the alveolar—arterial tension or diffusion gradient (A-a grad) and the arterial/alveolar tension ratio (a/A ratio). The A-a grad is simply the difference between the PAO_2 determined by the alveolar air equation and the PaO_2 determined by taking an arterial blood sample (gas) (an ABG). The a/A ratio is determined by dividing the PaO_2 by the PAO_2. An acceptable A-a grad on room air is a value less than 25 mmHg. An acceptable A-a grad on 100% oxygen is a value less than 125 mmHg. A normal value for the A-a grad varies as the FIO_2 changes. This makes it difficult to assess an acceptable value unless all the acceptable values are known for all FIO_2s. The acceptable value for the a/A ratio is greater than 0.75 for the complete range of FIO_2s. This makes it much easier to assess a patient's oxygenation status since only one number needs to be remembered.

a/A Ratio and A-a Gradient Calculations

For each of the above problems (9-5 to 9-12) where the PAO_2 was calculated, determine the A-a grad and the a/A ratio when given a PaO_2.

	PaO_2 (mmHg)	A-a Grad	a/A Ratio
9-13. PAO_2 of 9-5 ____	120	____	____
9-14. PAO_2 of 9-6 ____	550	____	____
9-15. PAO_2 of 9-7 ____	90	____	____
9-16. PAO_2 of 9-8 ____	60	____	____
9-17. PAO_2 of 9-9 ____	200	____	____
9-18. PAO_2 of 9-10 ____	70	____	____
9-19. PAO_2 of 9-11 ____	100	____	____
9-20. PAO_2 of 9-12 ____	150	____	____

PREDICTION OF REQUIRED FIO_2 AND RESULTANT PaO_2

Once an ABG is taken and an a/A ratio determined, it is possible to predict a resultant PaO_2 when the FIO_2 is changed. It is also possible to predict a required FIO_2 to achieve a desired PaO_2. The following formulas assume that the patient's $PaCO_2$ and lung condition have not changed.

Formula 1: Predicting a required FIO_2 to achieve a desired PaO_2.

Required FIO_2 = (desired PaO_2/a/A ratio + $PaCO_2$ × 1.25)/(Patm − 47)

Note: $PaCO_2$ × 1.25 is the same as $PaCO_2$/0.8 and, Patm − 47 is called the effective barometric pressure and will be labeled EBP.

Example

A patient is on a 30% air entrainment mask (AEM), has a PaO_2 of 50 mmHg, a $PaCO_2$ of 40 mmHg, and an a/A ratio of 0.31. The Patm is 747 mmHg. We want the patient to have a PaO_2 of 80 mmHg. What FIO_2 is required to achieve this goal?

Required FIO_2 = (desired PaO_2/a/A ratio + $PaCO_2$ × 1.25)/EBP

Required FIO_2 = (80/0.31 + 40 × 1.25)/700

Required FIO_2 = (258 + 50)/700 = 308/700 = 0.44 or 44%

Formula 2: Predicting a resultant PaO_2 with a given change of FIO_2.

Resultant PaO_2 = (EBP × new FIO_2 − $PaCO_2$ × 1.25) a/A ratio

---

Example

A patient is on mechanical ventilation and receiving 60% oxygen. The Patm is 760 mmHg. The patient's PaO_2 is 300 mmHg, his $PaCO_2$ is 50 mmHg and his a/A ratio is 0.82. If the maximum FIO_2 desired is 40%, what PaO_2 will result?

Resultant PaO_2 = (EBP × new FIO_2 − $PaCO_2$ × 1.25) a/A ratio

Resultant PaO_2 = (713 × 0.4 − 50 × 1.25) 0.82

Resultant PaO_2 = (285 − 62) 0.82 = 223 × 0.82 = 183 mmHg

Calculation of Required FIO_2 and Resultant PaO_2

Given the following information, calculate the required FIO_2 to achieve the desired PaO_2.

	Patm	FIO_2	PaO_2	$PaCO_2$	a/A	Desired PaO_2	Required FIO_2
9-21.	760	21	45	30	0.41	90	_____
9-22.	750	40	50	35	0.21	80	_____
9-23.	760	24	50	70	0.60	65	_____
9-24.	760	28	140	40	0.95	80	_____
9-25.	660	70	200	50	0.54	100	_____

Given the following information, calculate the resultant PaO_2 when the FIO_2 is changed.

	Patm	FIO_2	PaO_2	$PaCO_2$	a/A	FIO_2 Changed to	Resultant PaO_2 (mmHg)
9-26.	760	21	40	20	0.32	50	_____
9-27.	740	50	40	20	0.12	100	_____
9-28.	760	100	500	40	0.74	50	_____
9-29.	660	40	55	30	0.27	60	_____
9-30.	640	60	250	50	0.85	40	_____

For both sets of calculations above, the answers are estimates of actual results. There is no guarantee that the patient's cardiopulmonary status will remain the same, and patient changes will result in inaccurate calculations. The a/A ratio also, though rather stable throughout the change of FIO_2s, is not exact depending on the nature of the patient's problem. Still, the above calculations can be applied clinically with some good results.

OXYGEN CONTENT

The O_2 content of blood (arterial, CaO_2, or venous, CvO_2) is determined by the amount of O_2 dissolved in the plasma and the amount of O_2 carried on the hemoglobin (Hb).

Oxygen Dissolved in the Plasma

The amount of a gas dissolved in a liquid is determined by the partial pressure of the gas over the liquid, the temperature of the liquid, and the solubility of the gas in the liquid (Henry's Law). For determining CaO_2, blood is the liquid with a temperature of 37°C. The partial pressure of O_2 is the PaO_2, and the solubility coefficient for oxygen is 0.003 mL of oxygen per 100 mL of blood per millimeters of mercury pressure. The factor would appear as follows:

0.003 mL of O_2/dL blood/mmHg

(where dL = deciliter = 100 mL)

Examples

The following examples illustrate how this factor is used to determine the amount of O_2 dissolved in the blood.

Example A

$PaO_2 = 1$ mmHg;

1 mmHg $\times$ 0.003 mL O_2/dL/mmHg = 0.003 mL O_2/dL

Example B

$PaO_2 = 100$ mmHg;

100 mmHg $\times$ 0.003 mL O_2/dL/mmHg = 0.3 mL O_2/dL

Example C

$PaO_2 = 1000$ mmHg;

1000 mmHg $\times$ 0.003 mL O_2/dL/mmHg = 3.0 mL O_2/dL

NOTE: Example B is a "normal" PO_2, and example C is an example of a PO_2 under hyperbaric conditions. This is discussed in more detail in Chapter 14.

Dissolved Oxygen Content Calculations

Calculate the amount of O_2 dissolved in blood for the following PaO_2 values.

	PaO_2 (mmHg)	O_2 dissolved mL/dL Blood
9-31.	40	_____
9-32.	70	_____
9-33.	150	_____
9-34.	250	_____
9-35.	550	_____

Oxygen Carried on the Hemoglobin

At the molecular level, one molecule of hemoglobin (Hb) can carry four molecules of oxygen. If one molecule is attached, the Hb is 25% saturated; two molecules yield 50% saturation; three yield 75% saturation; and four yield 100% saturation. However, we do not measure at the molecular level but instead look at the grams (g) of Hb. One gram of Hb, when fully saturated, can carry 1.34 mL of oxygen. If 1 g Hb is carrying 0.335 mL of oxygen, it is 25% saturated; if 0.67 mL, then 50% saturated; if 1.005 mL, then 75% saturated; and at 1.34 mL, 100% saturated. The formula used to determine the amount of oxygen combined with Hb is expressed as follows:

---

grams of Hb $\times$ oxygen saturation $\times$ 1.34

Where:

grams of Hb is the g Hb/100 mL blood

oxygen saturation refers to "how full the Hb is filled" with oxygen compared with being totally filled (100%)

1.34 is the maximum amount of oxygen (in mL) that 1 g of Hb can hold when it is 100% saturated

---

Example 1
Calculate the amount of oxygen carried on Hb if the g of Hb = 14 and O_2Sat = 95%

$14 \times 0.95 \times 1.34 = 17.822$ mL of O_2 carried on Hb in 100 mL blood

---

Example 2
Calculate the amount of oxygen carried on Hb if the g of Hb = 10 and O_2Sat = 90%

$$10 \times 0.90 \times 1.34 = 12.06 \text{ mL } O_2/\text{dL blood}$$

Calculation of Oxygen Content on the Hemoglobin
Calculate the amount of oxygen carried on the Hb if given the following:

	Hb Grams	O_2 Sat	O_2 Carried on Hb mL/dL of Blood
9-36.	14	90	_____
9-37.	13	80	_____
9-38.	12	75	_____
9-39.	10	95	_____
9-40.	8	100	_____

Total Oxygen Content

To determine total oxygen content of arterial blood (CaO_2) or venous blood (CvO_2), the following formula is used.

$$O_2 \text{ content} = (0.003 \times PO_2) + (Hb \times O_2\text{Sat} \times 1.34)$$

Where:

0.003 is the solubility coefficient for O_2 in mL of O_2/dL of blood/mmHg.

PO_2 is the PO_2 in arterial blood (PaO_2) or the PO_2 in venous blood (PvO_2).

Hb is the grams (g) of Hb present in 100 mL of blood (g/dL mL) (g%).

O_2Sat is the saturation of Hb with O_2 (expressed here as a fraction).

1.34 is a constant, representing the maximum amount (mL) of O_2 that can be carried by 1 g of Hb (mL/g Hb) when Hb is 100% filled or saturated with oxygen. Note: Although 1.36 and 1.39 have been used in some texts for O_2 content determination, 1.34 will be used for this discussion.

O_2 content can be expressed in mL of O_2/100 mL of blood, or mL of O_2/dL of blood, or as volumes % (vol%).

Example A
For a "normal" individual with a PaO_2 of 100 mmHg, a Hb of 15 g, and a %Sat of 98%, the arterial O_2 content would be:

$$CaO_2 = (0.003 \times 100) + (15 \times 0.98 \times 1.34)$$
$$CaO_2 = 0.3 + 19.7 = 20.0 \text{ mL } O_2/\text{dL blood}$$

Example B
When breathing 100% O_2 at 1 Patm, the PaO_2 can reach levels as high as 600 mmHg. This has the potential of raising the CaO_2 somewhat, but content is limited because Hb is already 98% filled at a PaO_2 of 100 and the solubility coefficient is so low at 0.003.

$$CaO_2 = (0.003 \times 600) + (15 \times 1.0 \times 1.34)$$
$$CaO_2 = 1.8 + 20.1 = 21.9 \text{ mL } O_2/\text{dL blood}$$

Total Oxygen Content Calculations

Calculate the CaO_2 for the following conditions.

	PaO_2 (mmHg)	Hb (g)	O_2 Sat (%)	CaO_2 (mL O_2/dL blood)
9-41.	90	15	97	_____
9-42.	70	15	94	_____
9-43.	40	15	75	_____
9-44.	40	18	75	_____
9-45.	60	8	90	_____
9-46.	100	6	98	_____
9-47.	300	11	100	_____

A word concerning oxygen content. Normal CaO_2 is approximately 20 vol% and CvO_2 is 15 vol%. Sometimes we look at the 15 vol% as a reserve to draw from in case we get into trouble (develop hypoxemia). I would caution this notion. I think we need to consider O_2 content like we do a ladder. Which rungs are the most functional when attempting to clean leaves out of a house's gutters (spouting)? The answer is the upper rungs. (I know it depends on the size of the ladder and the height of the roof, but bear with me.) Then why do we have the lower rungs? Because their function is to get you to the upper rungs, but they have minimal function in allowing you to do your work once you are up. The 15 vol% of oxygen works the same way. We need the first 15 vol% to build on so that the top 5 vol% can be used. Some of the lower 15 vol% can be used as a reserve, but the lower its level, the less usable it is; therefore, it should only be thought of as a building block and not as a reserve. When the level drops too low, our cells become dysfunctional (let's say less than 50% sat). Even though there is a lot of oxygen present, it is not available for cellular use.

FRACTIONAL VERSUS FUNCTIONAL HEMOGLOBIN

Hemoglobin carries oxygen. The saturation of Hb is determined by the amount of oxygen carried on the Hb. Depending on how the calculation of oxygen saturation is determined, Hb actually may be carrying much less oxygen than it appears.

Fractional Hemoglobin

Fractional oxyhemoglobin (FO_2Hb) is the amount of oxyhemoglobin (O_2Hb) expressed as a fraction of the total hemoglobin (tHb). tHb includes all forms of Hb.

$$FO_2Hb = O_2Hb/tHb$$

Where:

$$tHb = O_2Hb + HHb + COHb + MetHb + ...$$

Because this calculation compares a part of the total Hb (oxyhemoglobin) with total Hb, it provides a more accurate indication of the amount of oxygen combined with Hb.

Functional Hemoglobin

Functional oxygen saturation, or oxygen saturation of available hemoglobin (SO_2), is the amount of oxyhemoglobin—expressed as a fraction of the Hb—that has the ability to bind with oxygen. This includes only oxyhemoglobin (O_2Hb) and deoxyhemoglobin (HHb). Sometimes HHb is incorrectly referred to as reduced Hb.

$$SO_2 = O_2Hb/(O_2Hb + HHb)$$

Because this calculation compares a part of the total Hb (oxyhemoglobin) with less than the total Hb, it does not provide an accurate indication of the amount of oxygen carried on the Hb. At times, a pa-

tient's FO_2Hb and SO_2 values may be very similar; at other times, they may be quite different.

Example 1
A patient has the following Hb levels (nonsmoker, rural dweller).

Hb Levels	Fraction of tHb	% of tHb
tHb = 12.0 g	1.0	100
O_2Hb = 11.28 g	0.94	94
COHb = 0.24 g	0.02	2
MetHb = 0.12 g	0.01	1
HHb = 0.36 g	0.03	3

$$FO_2Hb = 11.28/12 = .94 \text{ or } 94\%$$
$$SO_2 = 11.28/11.64 = .97 \text{ or } 97\%$$

Example 2
A patient has the following Hb levels (heavy smoker, city dweller).

Hb Levels	Fraction of tHb	% of tHb
tHb = 16.0 g	1.0	100
O_2Hb = 13.28 g	0.83	83
COHb = 1.6 g	0.1	10
MetHb = 0.48 g	0.03	3
HHb = 0.64 g	0.04	4

$$FO_2Hb = 13.28/16 = .83 \text{ or } 83\%$$
$$SO_2 = 13.28/13.92 = .95 \text{ or } 95\%$$

In example one, the two saturation values are similar. In example two, there is a great difference in the reported values. If the co-oximeter in use allows a choice between fractional and functional Hb readouts, choose the fractional setting. It gives a more accurate indication of the amount of O_2 actually present and available on the Hb.

Suggested Learning Activities

9-48. Spend time operating, calibrating, and in general, becoming familiar with a blood gas analyzer.

9-49. Blood gas analyzers can also measure the PO_2 and PCO_2 values in a gaseous sample. Inject a room air sample into the analyzer. Record the results. Are they the same as the predicted results? (Remember that the analyzer is calibrated to BTPS)

9-50. Using a blender, inject various percentages of oxygen gas sample into the analyzer. Record the results. Are they the same as predicted?

9-51. Bubble compressed air and 100% oxygen through water. Aspirate a water sample into a syringe and measure the PO_2 in the blood gas analyzer. Are they what you predicted? If not, why might they be different?

Oxyhemoglobin Dissociation Curve

PaO_2 and O_2Sat have a relationship expressed by the oxyhemoglobin (O_2Hb) dissociation curve. The graph of this curve, with O_2Sat on the Y axis and PaO_2 on the X axis, illustrates this relationship (Figure 9-1 in *Respiratory Care*). Owing to the binding nature of O_2 with Hb, the curve is sigmoid (S) shaped and not a straight line. Many factors can affect the relationship between these two variables. Some of these factors include $PaCO_2$, $[H^+]$ (hydrogen ion concentration), 2,3-diphosphoglycerate (2,3-DPG) levels, and patient temperature.

Increases in all of these factors will shift the curve to the right; decreases in these factors will shift the curve to the left. (Remember that increased $[H^+]$ will decrease pH). A right shift means that O_2 will not combine as readily with Hb but will be released by Hb more easily (decreased affinity). A left shift means that O_2 will combine very well with Hb but will not be released as well (increased affinity).

The actual amount of oxygen released to the tissues depends on many factors, and a blanket statement as to whether a right or left shift is "better" is inappropriate. A right shift results in a lower O_2Sat for any given PaO_2 compared with normal. A left shift results in a higher O_2Sat for any given PaO_2 compared with normal. For example, normally a PaO_2 of 60 mmHg will result in an O_2Sat of approximately 90%. A right shift, with a PaO_2 of 60 mmHg, would result in a lower saturation of <90%. A left shift, with a PaO_2 of 60 mmHg, would have a higher O_2Sat of >90%.

Many times, it can be determined if a curve is shifted right or left by knowing some normal relationships. A jingle I learned that I teach to my students is as follows: 30 is 60, 60 is 90, and 40 is 75. For a normal curve, a PaO_2 of 30 mmHg results in a saturation of 60%. A PaO_2 of 60 mmHg results in a saturation of 90%, and a PaO_2 of 40 mmHg results in 75% saturation. Of course normal P_{50} is 27 mmHg for Hb A as well. Knowing these few landmarks may help in determining if a curve is shifted right, left, or not at all.

Oxyhemoglobin Curve Shift Determination

Determine if the following are R shifts, L shifts, or No shift. Use Figure 9-1 in Respiratory Care *as a guide.*

	PaO_2 (mmHg)	O_2 sat (%)	Shift R-L-N
9-52.	60	95	_____
9-53.	60	85	_____
9-54.	40	70	_____
9-55.	40	80	_____
9-56.	55	90	_____
9-57.	45	75	_____
9-58.	80	92	_____
9-59.	70	98	_____
9-60.	27	50	_____

Determining whether a curve is shifted R or L may be more of an academic curiosity than a clinical necessity. It is more important to be able to determine oxygen content, oxygen delivery, and oxygen consumption than it is to know whether a curve is shifted R or L.

OXYGEN DELIVERY

Oxygen delivery (DO_2) is the amount of oxygen delivered by the arterial blood to the capillaries of the body for tissue use. The formula for DO_2 is:

$$DO_2 = CaO_2 \times CO$$

Where:

DO_2 is in mL O_2/min

CaO_2 is arterial oxygen content in mL O_2/100 mL blood

CO is cardiac output in mL/min

Note: The formula is often written: $DO_2 = CaO_2 \times CO \times 10$ where CaO_2 is mL O_2, CO is L/min, and 10 is a factor to convert everything to mL.

If normal CaO_2 is 20 mL/100 mL blood and normal CO is 5 L/min (5000 mL/min), then normal DO_2 equals:

$$DO_2 = 20 \text{ mL oxygen/100 mL blood} \times 5000 \text{ mL blood/min} = 1000 \text{ mL oxygen/min}$$

$$\text{(alternate form: } DO_2 = 20 \text{ mL} \times 5 \text{ L} \times 10 = 1000 \text{ mL)}$$

It is obvious from the formula that factors that affect CaO_2 or CO will also affect DO_2. This formula makes it easy to see why patients experiencing hypoxemia will have an increased CO to compensate for a low CaO_2, thereby attempting to restore DO_2. Routinely, it is desirable to keep DO_2 greater than 600 mL/min. If oxygen delivery falls below this value, tissue hypoxia is more likely to occur.

Oxygen Delivery Calculations

Determine the DO_2 of the following.

	CaO_2 (mL/dL)	CO (L/min)	DO_2 (mL/min)
9-61.	19.8	5	_____
9-62.	19.1	6	_____
9-63.	15.2	4	_____
9-64.	18.2	4	_____
9-65.	9.8	7	_____
9-66.	8.2	10	_____
9-67.	15.6	9	_____

OXYGEN CONSUMPTION

Oxygen consumption (VO_2) refers to the amount of oxygen leaving the capillaries that is consumed by the body's tissues. There are several ways to assess oxygen consumption. One method is calculation of the arterial-venous oxygen content difference (this is $CaO_2 - CvO_2$ or the a-v diff). Normal CaO_2 is 20 mL and normal CvO_2 is 15 mL. (CvO_2 must be measured in the pulmonary artery and not a peripheral vein.) The difference is 5 mL oxygen/100 mL blood. The a-v diff of 5 mL is the average amount of oxygen consumed by the tissues for every 100 mL of blood flowing through the body. Often it is desirable to measure the amount of VO_2 per minute. This can be done in two ways. The first is by using the a-v diff in the following formula:

$$VO_2 = \text{a-v diff} \times CO$$

$$VO_2 = 5 \text{ mL } O_2/100 \text{ mL blood} \times 5000 \text{ mL blood/min} \times 250 \text{ mL/min}$$

A second way to determine VO_2 is very similar to the above calculation, but is based on the difference between DO_2 and the O_2 returning to the heart (oxygen content in the venous system, CvO_2).

$$VO_2 = DO_2 - (CvO_2 \times CO)$$

$$VO_2 = 1000 \text{ mL } O_2/min - (15 \text{ mL } O_2/100 \text{ mL blood} \times 5000 \text{ mL blood/min})$$

$$VO_2 = 1000 \text{ mL } O_2/min - 750 \text{ mL } O_2/min = 250 \text{ mL } O_2/min$$

Normal VO_2 at rest is approximately 250 mL/min. During strenuous exercise, VO_2 can increase to 10 to 15 times the normal level. Stress factors (eg, trauma, infection, and fever) in hospital patients can also increase oxygen consumption.

OXYGEN EXTRACTION RATIO

The oxygen extraction ratio, or called by some the oxygen utilization coefficient (OUC), is a calculation of the amount of oxygen consumed compared with the amount of oxygen delivered to the tissues. It can be evaluated for every 100 mL of blood or for total oxygen delivery per minute. Both formulas are presented below.

$$\text{Based on a dL of blood: OUC} = (CaO_2 - CvO_2)/CaO_2$$

$$\text{OUC} = (20 - 15)/20 = 0.25$$

$$\text{Based on a minute: OUC} = VO_2/DO_2$$

$$\text{OUC} = 250/1000 = 0.25$$

The OUC value has no units because they cancel out in the formula. Both of these methods require a fair amount of data collecting and calculation. A quick estimate of the OUC can be obtained by looking at the oxygen saturation of both arterial and venous blood. This method is acceptable, since most of the oxygen content is carried on the hemoglobin.

$$OUC = (SaO_2 - SvO_2)/SaO_2$$
$$OUC = (98 - 75)/98 = 0.235$$

This value can be continuously monitored if a patient has both an arterial saturation monitor and an indwelling venous saturation monitoring device. Normal values for OUC are less than 0.35. For values greater than 0.35, concerns should be raised. One of the concerns could be that CO is not sufficient. Another concern is that metabolism (oxygen consumption) has increased significantly.

Calculation of VO$_2$ and OUC

Calculate the following:

	CaO$_2$ (mL)	CvO$_2$ (mL)	CO (L/min)	VO$_2$ (mL/min)	OUC
9-68.	20	15	7	_____	_____
9-69.	15	10	6	_____	_____
9-70.	17	14	10	_____	_____
9-71.	13	7	4	_____	_____
9-72.	20	13	15	_____	_____

ABG INTERPRETATION

Individuals, when introduced to ABG interpretation, can find it fun or frustrating. I would stress three main areas when interpreting ABGs. The first is that you must know the normal values. Next, you must keep the relationship between pH, PaCO$_2$, and HCO$_3$ straight. Last, you must be systematic in your approach. Normal values for arterial and venous blood are found in Table 9-1.

TABLE 9-1 **Normal Values for Arterial and Venous Blood Samples***

	Arterial*	Venous*
pH	7.40	7.37
PCO$_2$	40	46
PO$_2$	90	40
O$_2$Sat	97	75
BE	0	0
HCO$_3$	24	24

*There is, of course, a range of normals, but this one set of values will do as a reference point.

Relationship Between pH, PCO$_2$, and HCO$_3$

As PCO$_2$ goes up or as HCO$_3$ goes down, pH goes down. As PCO$_2$ goes down or as HCO$_3$ goes up, pH goes up. Another way of putting it is to say that pH is directly proportional to HCO$_3$ and inversely proportional to PCO$_2$. Remember from the Henderson-Hasselbach equation that:

$$pH \propto HCO_3/(PCO_2 \times 0.03) \text{ at a ratio of } 24:1.2$$
$$\text{or } 20:1$$

Even if HCO$_3$ and PCO$_2$ change, but the ratio stays 20:1, pH remains 7.40. If the ratio is greater than 20:1, then alkalemia occurs. If the ratio is less than 20:1, acidemia occurs.

Systematic Interpretation

You may use any system that works for you. If you do not have one, I recommend the following.

1. Look at the pH. Is it increased, decreased, or normal?
2. Look at the PCO$_2$. Is it normal or abnormal? If abnormal, is it contributing to the pH problem or compensating for it?
3. Look at the HCO$_3$. Is it normal or abnormal? If abnormal, is it contributing to the pH problem or compensating for it?
4. Look at the PaO$_2$. Is it increased, decreased, or normal?
5. Look at the FiO$_2$. Is it room air or increased?

Example A

$$pH = 7.30; PCO_2 = 54; HCO_3 = 25; BE = +1; PaO_2 = 55; FIO_2 = 21\%$$

1. pH is decreased; acidemia
2. $PaCO_2$ is increased; respiratory acidemia
3. HCO_3 is normal; no compensation
4. PaO_2 is decreased; hypoxemia
5. FIO_2 is room air

Interpretation: uncompensated respiratory acidemia with hypoxemia on room air

Example B

$$pH = 7.54; PCO_2 = 32; HCO_3 = 29; BE = +5; PaO_2 = 120; FIO_2 = 40\%$$

1. pH is increased; alkalemia
2. $PaCO_2$ is decreased; respiratory alkalemia
3. HCO_3 is increased; metabolic alkalemia
4. PaO_2 is increased; hyperoxemia
5. FIO_2 is 40%

Interpretation: combined (mixed) respiratory and metabolic alkalemia with hyperoxemia on 40% oxygen

Example C

$$pH = 7.33; PCO_2 = 60; HCO_3 = 29; BE = +5; PaO_2 = 80; FIO_2 = 30\%$$

1. pH is decreased; acidemia
2. $PaCO_2$ is increased; respiratory acidemia
3. HCO_3 is increased; compensating
4. PaO_2 is normal
5. FIO_2 is 30%

Interpretation: partially compensated respiratory acidemia with adequate oxygenation on 30% oxygen

Example D

$$pH = 7.32; PCO_2 = 34; HCO_3 = 17; BE = -7; PaO_2 = 90; FIO_2 = 21\%$$

1. pH is decreased; acidemia
2. $PaCO_2$ is decreased; compensating
3. HCO_3 is decreased; metabolic acidemia
4. PaO_2 is normal
5. FIO_2 is 21%

Interpretation: partially compensated metabolic acidemia with adequate oxygenation on room air

ABG Interpretation

Interpret the following ABGs.

	pH	PaCO$_2$	HCO$_3$	BE	PaO$_2$	FIO$_2$
9-73.	7.06	12	2	−35	125	0.21
9-74.	7.24	75	32	+8	60	0.30
9-75.	7.48	30	24	0	85	0.21
9-76.	7.32	32	15	−8	55	0.40
9-77.	7.49	44	21	−3	120	0.21
9-78.	7.40	50	29	+5	70	0.50
9-79.	7.50	80	50	+25	300	1.00
9-80.	7.44	55	37	+12	45	0.24

ACID-BASE CALCULATIONS AND EXERCISES

When the body experiences an acid-base disturbance, it will respond in the following manner.

1. Buffering will occur. The body's buffers will buffer each other. This starts to happen very quickly (seconds) and attempts to minimize a pH change.
2. Compensation will occur (if possible). If the problem is metabolic, the respiratory system will quickly (minutes) respond and attempt to minimize pH change (eg, diabetic ketoacidosis). If the problem is respiratory, the metabolic system (kidneys) will slowly respond (hours to days) to minimize pH change (eg, COPD). In mild cases, compensation *may* be complete (fully compensated) and bring the pH back to normal. In more severe cases, each of these systems, if pushed to their limits, will reach a point of maximum compensation (they can do no more), but the acid-base disorder itself will only be partially compensated.
3. Correction will occur (if possible). The primary system causing the disorder will start to correct the imbalance. In severe cases where the body

cannot correct the problem, the correction process is often aided by medical personnel. Mechanical ventilation is initiated for the acute ventilatory failure patient. Sodium bicarbonate is given to the patient with severe metabolic acidosis.

Being able to interpret ABG reports is fun and challenging, but knowing what the values mean and how to deal with abnormal results is much more important.

Heparin Dilution

Along with the changes mentioned in *Respiratory Care*, dilution of blood with heparinized solutions can also change HCO_3, BE, and hemoglobin values dramatically. It is important to remember that if significant heparin dilution is suspected, the results from the analysis of the sample are totally invalid, and the blood sample must be obtained again. A formula to estimate the effect of dilution on both $PaCO_2$ and Hb is as follows:

Actual Hb = Measured Hb ×
$$[1+ (mL_1/(mL_2 - mL_1))]$$

Actual $PaCO_2$ = Measured $PaCO_2$ ×
$$[1+ (mL_1/(mL_2 - mL_1))]$$

Where:

mL_1 is the volume of heparinized solution in the sample

mL_2 is the total volume of the sample

These calculations can be done because the heparinized solution has no Hb and very little CO_2. In both cases, a physical dilution occurs, like mixing water with orange juice, where the orange juice becomes more dilute. This same process cannot predict changes in pH, HCO_3, or PaO_2. This same type of effect would occur with other diluents as well; however, just heparinized solutions are discussed here because they are used with ABG samples to prevent clotting of blood.

Research Project

9-80. Perform an experiment diluting blood with a heparinized solution at various ratios of mixture of heparin solution and blood. Analyze the samples. Determine if the above formulas can predict the changes in Hb and $PaCO_2$. More importantly, note how heparin dilution causes the sample results to be inaccurate.

BLOOD SAMPLE EXERCISES

Obtaining Arterial Blood Samples

An artery is a pressurized vessel. If a needle punctures that pressurized vessel, blood will come out, regardless of the needle's angle or direction of insertion. (I have, on occasion, had to stick an artery in the opposite direction and even upside down.) There is, however, an accepted procedure for performing arterial punctures, and this procedure should be followed whenever possible. This procedure is described in *Respiratory Care*. I would not recommend the routine use of Xylocaine on patients. I would reserve it for the very difficult patient situations. In my 20 years of practice, I have obtained and helped students obtain well over 10,000 blood gas samples. I have only ever used Xylocaine two times.

Critical Thinking Exercises

You are a night shift respiratory care practitioner and obtained several ABGs from peripheral vessels. The physician in charge of the patients, challenges you as to whether these are arterial or venous samples. In no cases were the samples mixed (part arterial and part venous). Which of the following blood samples (9-81 through 9-84) *could be* arterial? Venous? How do you know? What other factors can be evaluated to help in the differentiation?
  (Check answer key.)

9-81. pH = 7.44 PCO_2 = 37 HCO_3 = 25 PO_2 = 70 O_2Sat = 95%

9-82. pH = 7.35 PCO_2 = 42 HCO_3 = 22 PO_2 = 55 O_2Sat = 88%

9-83. pH = 7.30 PCO_2 = 46 HCO_3 = 20 PO_2 = 40 O_2Sat = 75%

9-84. pH = 7.40 PCO_2 = 30 HCO_3 = 19 PO_2 = 40 O_2Sat = 75%

9-85. A normal person with normal metabolism, CO_2, and so forth, is breathing 100% oxygen. His PaO_2 is 600 mmHg and Hb is 14 g%. What will his venous oxygen (PvO_2) be? Pick a number from below, then try to calculate the answer. (Check answer key in back of text.)

40, 50, 90, 150, 300, 450, or 540 mmHg

10

Fiberoptic Bronchoscopy

Bronchoscopy is a safe and beneficial procedure. Bronchoscopy may be performed in many settings, including those done on an outpatient bases or in the critical care setting. Teaching scopes are available that have a second eyepiece so an observer can watch. Appropriate systems can also be set up to allow the image to be displayed on a monitor for better viewing.

CASE STUDY

T. S. was a 38-year-old white female weighing 200 pounds. She had an unremarkable medical history and had been in good health. In October, after inhaling dust while on a hayride, she experienced a severe coughing/choking episode and had trouble getting her breath. Following the acute episode, she developed a mild but persistent cough. Three months later, in January, the cough became worse and wheezing was present in her right lung. She had no expectoration or hemoptysis and no history of asthma or respiratory allergies. She did have a 30-pack/year smoking history. In April, her family doctor referred her to a pulmonologist. At this time, she complained of increased chest tightness, wheezing, and coughing. She was not short of breath. Her complete blood count and total eosinophiles were normal. Pulmonary function tests were done, which showed normal volumes and flows except for a very mild decrease in forced expiratory flow $(FEF)_{25-75}$. Following a short trial of oral steroids and metered-dose inhaler bronchodilator therapy with no improvement, a bronchoscopy was performed to rule out foreign body presence. The bronchoscopy revealed a normal evaluation with no evidence of any foreign bodies. Two weeks later with no improvement, a methacholine challenge study was conducted. This test proved negative for bronchial reactivity. A repeat chest radiograph was also negative for any abnormalities. T. S. was then started on antimicrobial therapy and bronchodilators. Her symptoms improved over the next month but persisted. A barium swallow was ordered to rule out reflux or aspiration. The results were normal without indication of reflux or aspiration. A computed tomography study of the thorax was obtained. The results were negative for mediastinal mass or adenopathy. There were some streaky densities at both bases, which could have represented atelectasis or an inflammatory process. Over the next few months, the patient continued to improve, and although a mild cough persisted, the wheezing diminished. Then, in June (20 months after the initial episode), the patient's symptoms became worse with increased coughing and wheezing on the right. A second bronchoscopy was scheduled to re-evaluate the airway. The left lung bronchi appeared normal, as did the right upper and middle lobe bronchi. The right lower lobe bronchus, however, had marked mucosal edema and inflammation with significant compromise of the lumen. Within the lumen a gray-yellow object was noted. Retrieval by forceps revealed a 3-cm-long piece of straw. The patient was given antimicrobial therapy. Over the next weeks, the patient's symptoms gradually improved and T. S. became asymptomatic 22 months after the hayride.

STUDENT EXERCISES

10-1. List five common diagnostic indications for a bronchoscopy.

a. _____

b. _____

c. _____

d. _____

e. _____

10-2. List five therapeutic indications for a bronchoscopy.

a. _____

b. _____

c. _____

d. _____

e. _____

10-3. List two contraindications to bronchoscopy.

a. _____

b. _____

10-4. List five relative contraindications to bronchoscopy.

a. _____

b. _____

c. _____

d. _____

e. _____

10-5. List the six diagnostic procedures performed with fiberoptic bronchoscopy.

a. _____

b. _____

c. _____

d. _____

e. _____

f. _____

REVIEW QUESTIONS

10-6. The most common indication for a bronchoscopic procedure is which of the following?
A. hemoptysis
B. chest pain
C. abnormal roentgenographic study
D. excessive sputum production

10-7. Which of the following are correct concerning the use of the bronchoscope?
A. foreign bodies in the airway can almost always be removed with the bronchoscope.
B. bronchoalveolar lavage is routinely used in an attempt to diagnose infection
C. a lung abscess is a strong indication for bronchoscopy
D. all of the above

10-8. The most frequent therapeutic use of the bronchoscope is which of the following?
A. remove retained secretions
B. check endotracheal tube placement
C. remove foreign bodies
D. laser therapy

10-9. Which of the following would not be listed as a complication of bronchoscopic evaluation?
A. hypoxemia
B. hypocarbia
C. hypotension
D. bradycardia

10-10. The hypopharynx should be anesthetized with which of the following?
A. 2.25% epinephrine
B. 5% atropine
C. 2% lidocaine
D. 2 puffs of vanceril

10-11. Cleaning the bronchoscope may involve all of the following except:
A. rinsing it with saline after use
B. soaking in glutaraldehyde
C. use of an autoclave
D. use of gas sterilization

11

Sleep-Disordered Breathing

Sleep—what is it? What happens when we sleep? How much sleep do we need? These and other questions regarding sleep continue to be addressed as more and more is known about this mysterious subject. The ways in which sleep, or lack of it, influences our lives is also being studied. The study of sleep disorders may be one of the fastest growing and most fascinating areas of medicine.

KEY TERMS AND DEFINITIONS

Apneic event: Cessation of breathing (air movement) for 10 seconds or longer.

Hypopneic event: A decrease in volume during tidal breathing to levels of one half of baseline volumes for 8 seconds or longer.

Apnea/hypopnea index: The average number of apneic and hypopneic events per hour of sleep. The upper limit of normal is 10/h.

Desaturation event: A decrease in oxygen saturation of more than 4% from the baseline reading.

CASE STUDIES

Case Study 1

C. H. is a 12-year-old girl. She is 65 inches tall and weighs 200 lb.

History

Her medical history is unremarkable. She is taking no medications and has no known allergies (NKA). On examination, her pulse was 82, SpO_2 of 96% at rest on room air, lungs clear, and her tonsils were enlarged. She does experience shortness of breath (SOB) walking up two flights of stairs.

Sleep Note

Although she wakes from sleep feeling rested, she experiences daytime hypersomnolence (sleepiness) and morning headaches. C. H. has been observed on occasion to sit up in bed, with SOB, during the night and does snore while sleeping.

Results of Nocturnal Polysomnography (Sleep Study)

apnea/hypopnea index = 53/h
mean duration of apnea = 17 seconds
significant arterial desaturation with a low of 46%
mean saturation during apneic events, 79%

Results of Sleep Study With Nasal Continuous Positive Airway Pressure (nCPAP) at 10 cmH$_2$O:

apnea/hypopnea index = 8/h
lowest Sat = 82%
mean Sat during apneic events = 88%

Conclusions

Patient is experiencing significant obstructive apnea, hypopnea, and arterial desaturation while sleeping. There was significant improvement with use of 10 cmH$_2$O nCPAP. Apneic events decreased from 23/h to 3/h. Lowest oxygen saturation increased from 46% to 82%.

Recommendations

nCPAP at 10 cmH$_2$O at night
possible tonsillectomy
weight reduction

Case Study 2

D. G. is a 52-year-old man. He is 70 inches tall and weighs 195 lb.

History

D. G. is a well-nourished, well-developed man who presented alert and in no apparent distress. Patient is hypertensive with a blood pressure of 142/90. His lungs were clear and a peak flow (PF) was 550 L/min. There was no jugular vein distention, and cardiac rhythm was regular. Patient denies smoking, drinking, and using sedatives. Patient does experience mild dyspnea on exertion. He had surgery for correction of a deviated nasal septum. Patient states that he feels he has had some personality changes recently.

Sleep Note

D. G. awakes from sleep feeling tired in the morning. He complains of morning headaches and daytime sleepiness. He has fallen asleep while driving and in the middle of conversations. His condition does not interfere with his job. He has had frequent and heavy snoring and snorting for many years. This wakes him at night. He also develops SOB and feels like he is gasping for air at night. His wife has reported that he has periods of apnea and mild kicking and thrashing while sleeping. He repositions himself often at night. He also complains of nasal congestion and of his throat bothering him, like it is closing up.

Results of Sleep Study

Patient had 227 apneas with an apnea/hypopnea index of 70/h.

There were 116 desaturation events with the lowest recorded at 74%.

There was loud snoring/snorting as well as gasping types of respirations.

There was mild leg movement and frequent turning.

Results of Sleep Study With nCPAP at 14 cmH$_2$O

apnea/hypopnea index = 5/h
no desaturation events

Conclusions

Patient has significant obstructive sleep apnea (OSA) with desaturation. Significant improvement with nCPAP at 14 cmH$_2$O.

Recommendation

nCPAP at 14 cmH$_2$O while sleeping

Follow-Up

D. G. elected not to use CPAP but pursued a surgical option. He underwent a uvulopalatopharyngoplasty and a hyoid suspension. Three months later, he also underwent a septoplasty and turbinate resection. Following these procedures, the patient's condition was much improved.

Case Study 3

H. B. is a 42-year-old man. He is 65 inches tall with morbid obesity at 425 lb.

History

The patient presented alert and in no apparent distress. He has mild hypertension with a blood pressure of 142/88. His oxygen saturation is 88% to 92% on room air at rest. He complains of some nasal congestion and dyspnea on exertion. Patient examination reveals a crowed pharynx and decreased breath sounds. There is no clubbing, edema, or cyanosis present. Patient denies a history of smoking, drink-

ing, or using sedatives. He does state that at times he has some mental confusion.

Sleep Note

H. B. stated he feels tired in the morning and has morning headaches. During the day, he experiences excessive daytime sleepiness. He has drowsiness while driving, during meetings, and while conversing with others. He also falls asleep while visiting friends. At night he has frequent heavy snoring and snorting. He gasps for air and has SOB. Apneic spells are reported by his wife for as long as 30 seconds. He awakens frequently at night, has many position changes, and displays severe kicking and thrashing.

Results of Sleep Test

apnea/hypopnea index = 113/h

mean duration of apnea = 14.4 seconds

mean duration of hypopnea = 14.8 seconds

patient had 674 desaturation events with the lowest recorded at 32%

The entire night was spent at less than 90% sat.

There was loud snoring and excessive limb movement.

Gasping respirations were also noted.

The patient stated, "I had a normal night's sleep."

Results of Sleep Test With 15 cmH$_2$O

Apnea and hypopnea were still present with some snoring and frequent awakenings.

There were 197 desaturation events with the lowest at 62%.

Three liters of oxygen via nasal cannula was added to the CPAP to maintain oxygen saturations above 86% during sleep.

Patient demonstrated mild leg and arm movements.

Conclusions

Patient is experiencing severe OSA with very significant apnea, hypopnea, and arterial oxygen desaturation. There is a decreased severity with the use of nCPAP and supplemental oxygen.

Recommendations

Use of nCPAP at night along with 3 L/min cannula. If patient does not improve on nCPAP, or if the patient does not tolerate it, a tracheostomy will be considered. It was highly recommended that the patient lose weight.

Follow-Up

After 3 months of use, the patient refused to use the CPAP, finding it intolerable, even though it had given some relief of symptoms. The patient will be given a trial on bilevel positive airway pressure (BiPAP). If he does not tolerate this, a trach will again be considered.

Case Study 4

J. B. is a 43-year-old man. He is 67 inches tall with massive obesity at 385 lb. (J. B. is the older brother of H. B. in Case Study 3.)

History

J. B. has hypertension with a blood pressure of 145/90. On examination, his pulse was 72, respirations 14 and unlabored, and breath sounds clear. He denies smoking or using sedatives. He is an occasional drinker. J. B. has a very small oropharynx with excess tissue present and a large tongue. He had a tonsillectomy and adenoidectomy as a child. He presents with 2+ pitting edema up to the knees, but no cyanosis is present. He does report a decreased attention span.

Sleep Note

He reports that he feels tired in the morning following sleep. He does not have morning headaches, but his legs do hurt. He has daytime somnolence. This expresses itself during conversation with others and while he is standing at a desk at work. This sleepiness does interfere with his work, and his supervisor has brought it to his attention. He has fallen asleep while driving, and one time ran into a school bus. At night, he occasionally snores loudly and has been for 15 years. His father-in-law has told him he stops breathing at night (>15 seconds) at their hunting camp. Gasping has also been reported at night. J. B. does not kick and thrash at night, but he does change position frequently. He likes to have a fan blowing air over him at night or else he feels like he is choking.

Results of Sleep Study

apnea/hypopnea index = 67/h

significant desaturations with a low of 62%

209 desaturations with a mean of 82% during the apneic events

patient exhibited loud snoring, some leg movement, and bradycardia with events

Results of Sleep Study on nCPAP at 15 cmH$_2$O

At 15 cmH$_2$O nCPAP, the patient still experienced some apnea and hypopnea. Snoring was eliminated at 10 cmH$_2$O. The apnea/hypopnea index was 5/h, and the arterial saturations did not drop below 90%. There was no excessive limb movement. The patient commented that he slept better, felt more rested, and his legs did not hurt.

Conclusions

Patient has significant OSA with marked improvement while using nCPAP. Apnea/hypopnea index decreasing from 67 to 5 and saturations increasing from a low of 62% to a low of 90%.

Recommendations

Use of nCPAP while sleeping at 15 cmH$_2$O
Weight reduction

Follow-Up

One month later, J. B. returned to the doctor stating that "I feel like a new man." He wakes up refreshed and ready to go. He has increased energy and his family is very happy.

REVIEW QUESTIONS

11-1. It has been estimated that fatigue is a factor in what percent of accidents leading to the death of truck drivers?
   A. 2%
   B. 13%
   C. 34%
   D. 57%

11-2. All of the following are true concerning slow wave sleep except:
   A. increased upper airway resistance
   B. growth hormone is secreted
   C. there is an increase in minute ventilation
   D. arterial carbon dioxide increases 3 to 7 mmHg

11-3. Snoring has been associated with each of the following except:
   A. hypertension
   B. lung cancer
   C. stroke
   D. heart disease

11-4. severity of snoring is increased with each of the following except:
   A. supine position
   B. weight gain
   C. smoking
   D. use of alcohol

11-5. Each of the following are associated with OSA except:
   A. decreased blood pressure
   B. decreased heart rate
   C. decreased cardiac output
   D. decreased SaO$_2$

11-6. Each of the following are symptoms of OSA except:
   A. intellectual deterioration
   B. morning headache
   C. impotency
   D. hypotension

11-7. All of the following have been shown to reduce the severity of sleep apnea except:
   A. weight loss
   B. eliminating alcohol consumption
   C. decreasing cigarette smoking
   D. changing sleeping position

11-8. Common side effects of CPAP used for treatment of OSA include each of the following except:
  A. sore eyes
  B. dry mouth
  C. rhinorrhea
  D. diminished sense of smell

11-9. All of the following are true concerning central sleep apnea except:
  A. it occurs exclusively during rapid eye movement sleep
  B. it is much less common than OSA
  C. patients tend to be older
  D. it is often secondary to other medical disorders

11-10. Use of which of the following medications has shown improvement in the treatment of central sleep apnea?
  A. theophylline
  B. medroxyprogesterone acetate
  C. acetazolamide
  D. triazolam

12

Respiratory Care Monitoring

LABORATORY EXERCISES: PULSE OXIMETRY

12-1. Obtain two pulse oximeters and compare their readings on several volunteers. Do they yield the same readings? Does one consistently read higher than the other?

12-2. Using the normal oxyhemoglobin dissociation curve, estimate the PO_2 based on the following oxygen saturations.

	O_2Sat (%)	PO_2 (mmHg)
a.	90	_____
b.	80	_____
c.	75	_____
d.	50	_____
e.	97	_____
f.	85	_____
g.	93	_____

12-3. Using the normal oxyhemoglobin dissociation curve, estimate the O_2Sat based on the following PO_2s.

	PO_2 (mmHg)	O_2Sat (%)
a.	120	_____
b.	100	_____
c.	80	_____
d.	65	_____
e.	50	_____
f.	45	_____
g.	30	_____

LABORATORY EXERCISES: HEMODYNAMIC PARAMETERS

For each of the following calculations, use the formulas presented in Respiratory Care, *Table 12-4.*

12-4. **Given:**

SBP = 120 mmHg	DBP = 80 mmHg
SPAP = 28 mmHg	DPAP = 12 mmHg
CO = 5.6 L/min	BSA = 2 M²
HR = 80 beats/min	
CVP = 5 mmHg	PCWP = 10 mmHg

Calculate:

MAP = _____ mmHg
MPAP = _____ mmHg
CI = _____
SV = _____ mL
PVR = _____ dynes-sec/cm⁵
SVR = _____ dynes-sec/cm⁵

12-5. **Given:**

SBP = 140 mmHg	DBP = 90 mmHg
SPAP = 45 mmHg	DPAP = 25 mmHg
CO = 9.0 L/min	BSA = 2.5 M²
HR = 120 beats/min	
CVP = 10 mmHg	PCWP = 15 mmHg

Calculate:

MAP = _____ mmHg
MPAP = _____ mmHg
CI = _____
SV = _____ mL
PVR = _____ dynes-sec/cm⁵
SVR = _____ dynes-sec/cm⁵

CALORIMETRY

Calorimetry is a method used to measure energy expenditure or metabolic rate. Direct calorimetry accomplishes this by measuring heat production. Indirect calorimetry determines energy expenditure by measuring VO_2 and VCO_2. The Weir Equation allows the calculation of calorie usage based on VO_2 and VCO_2. The open-circuit technique determines VO_2 and VCO_2 by measuring exhaled gas concentrations and minute ventilation. From these measurements, the respiratory quotient (RQ) (VCO_2/VO_2) can also be calculated.

Laboratory Exercises: Indirect Calorimetry

For each of the following calculations, use formulas presented in Respiratory Care, *Equation Box 1, Chapter 12.*

12-6. **Given:**

VO_2 = 250 mL/min
VCO_2 = 200 mL/min

Calculate:

The estimated REE based on the VO_2 only _____ kcal/day
The estimated REE based on the VCO_2 only _____ kcal/day
The REE based on the Weir equation _____ kcal/day
The RQ _____

12-7. **Given:**

V_E = 8.6 L/min V_I = 8.6 L/min
$FICO_2$ = 0.0003 $FECO_2$ = 0.041
FIO_2 = 0.21 FEO_2 = 0.17

Calculate:

The REE based on the Weir equation _____ kcal/day
The RQ _____

VOLUME LOSS DUE TO COMPRESSION

When patients are being mechanically ventilated, some of the set volume is never delivered to the patient's airway. During inspiration, when the system is pressurized, gas is compressed in the circuit. This compressed gas accounts for what is known as "volume loss due to compression." This volume loss (VL) robs the patient of alveolar ventilation, and delivered minute ventilation will need to be increased to compensate. (Remember that required minute ventilation is usually documented by arterial blood gas [ABG] analysis.) Several factors affect the amount of volume loss. These include length and volume of the tubing and humidifier system, tubing compliance, and system pressure and temperature.

Calculation of volume loss due to compression should involve a two-step procedure. The first step involves the calculation of the compression factor (Cf), which is really the compliance of the patient circuit. This is accomplished by one of two methods. The first method begins with the ventilator and tubing completely assembled, and the patient connection capped. Set a volume on the ventilator of 100 to 200 mL. Set the pressure limit at its maximum. Adjust the flow rate to a very low value, and cycle the ventilator. The machine will volume cycle. Observe the peak inspiratory pressure (PIP) for the delivered volume. The second method also begins with the ventilator and tubing completely assembled, and the patient con-

nection capped. Set a desired pressure limit at 40 to 80 cmH_2O. Set the VT at 500 mL. Adjust the flow rate to a very low value, and cycle the ventilator. The machine will pressure cycle. Observe the delivered volume at the pressure limit. Using either method, the Cf is now determined by using the following formula:

$$Cf = delivered\ VT/(PIP - EEP)$$

Where:

Cf is the compression factor or the compliance of the patient circuit for a given set of conditions (mL/cmH_2O)
VT is the volume used to pressurize the circuit (mL)
PIP is peak inspiratory pressure (cmH_2O)
EEP is the end expiratory or baseline pressure (cmH_2O)

Example

A 150-mL volume is compressed into a capped circuit at a pressure of 50 cmH_2O. No PEEP is present. The Cf is calculated by dividing 150 mL/50 cmH_2O, equaling 3 mL/cm H_2O. The Cf is the number of mL of gas that will be trapped in the circuit for every 1 cmH_2O pressure applied to the system. The Cf will typically fall between 1.5 and 3 mL/cmH_2O for adult circuits, but will vary from circuit to circuit and at different system pressures.

The second step in determining the actual VL is to multiply the compression factor times the actual system pressure during patient ventilation using the following formula:

$$Cf \times PIP = VL$$

Example

A patient is being ventilated and the PIP is 40 cmH_2O. The circuit Cf is measured at 3 mL/cmH_2O. The VL is calculated by multiplying Cf × PIP = 3 × 40 = 120 mL. If a VT of 700 mL is delivered from the ventilator, only 580 mL (700 − 120) reaches the patient airway. The 580 mL represents the corrected VT and should be used for compliance calculations. If the patient has a dead space (VD) of 180 mL, only 400 mL (580 − 180) comprises alveolar ventilation per breath. Note that some mechanical ventilators now have the ability to automatically compensate for VL and adjust the delivered VT appropriately. This option will instruct the ventilator to deliver extra volume to compensate for the volume loss, and it will not be shown as part of the exhaled volume reading.

Measuring Volume Loss Due to Compression

VL due to compression can be determined by measuring exhaled gas at two different sites and determining the difference. One site is at the exhalation valve. The other site is at the endotracheal tube, in the mechanical dead space. By measuring the volumes at both sites and determining the difference, the VL is calculated. Ventilators that have a continuous flow of gas through the circuit may not yield accurate readings.

Laboratory Exercises

12-8. Using a ventilator and circuit, determine the compliance of the patient circuit. Repeat this exercise for different circuits and at several pressure levels. Record the results.

12-9. Set up a mechanical ventilator in the A/C mode and attach it to a test lung. Deliver a set VT and measure the volume exiting the exhalation port. Also measure the volume exiting from the test lung. A Wright respirometer or similar device can be used. The difference between the two values is the VL due to compression. Calculate the VL due to compression based on the compression factor of the circuit. Compare the measured VL with the calculated VL.

AUTO-PEEP

Auto-positive end-expiratory pressure (auto-PEEP) is present when there is an EEP greater than the set baseline pressure at end exhalation. Auto-PEEP occurs when expiratory time (TE) is too short to allow complete exhalation to baseline pressure level. Patient factors, such as compliance and resistance, must also be considered. Auto-PEEP results in increased trapped gas volume in the patient's lungs. Auto-PEEP is an index of that trapped volume. Years ago, this was documented on patients, especially those with chronic obstructive pulmonary disease (COPD). Following an inspiration, the rate control was temporarily turned down so that a breath would not be delivered. The Bennett spirometer would continue to rise several hundred milliliters above the set VT. This extra volume was trapped air, auto-PEEP, but no one termed it as such at that time. This technique may still work in some ventilators.

The actual amount of volume retained in the lungs by PEEP or auto-PEEP can be calculated if the patient's static compliance (Cst) is known by using the following formula:

Retained (or trapped) volume = Cst × total PEEP

Example

A patient has a Cst of 30 mL/cmH$_2$O. His PEEP level is +10 cmH$_2$O. His functional residual capacity (FRC) has been increased by 300 mL by the +10 of PEEP;

30 mL/cmH$_2$O × 10 cmH$_2$O = 300 mL

Following some ventilator parameter changes, the patient is experiencing auto-PEEP with a total PEEP level of +15 cmH$_2$O. If his compliance is still 30 mL/cmH$_2$O, his total trapped volume is 450 mL;

30 mL/cmH$_2$O × 15 cmH$_2$O = 450 mL

The auto-PEEP is causing an extra 150 mL of volume to be trapped in his lung.

Laboratory Exercise

12-10. Using a mechanical ventilator and a test lung, create auto-PEEP. Begin with normal ventilation parameters. Then, by increasing the respiratory frequency or increasing inspiratory time (increase VT or decrease flow), cause the TE to become very short. Using a Braschi valve or a ventilator with an expiratory hold, measure the amount of auto-PEEP created. Try using a test lung where resistance and compliance can be adjusted and repeat the study.

There are some important items that should be pointed out concerning auto-PEEP. (1) Auto-PEEP can only be measured accurately when the patient is resting and not actively breathing. (2) Resistance × Compliance equals what is known as a time constant. Different areas of the lungs have different resistance and compliance or time constant values. This means that auto-PEEP level or trapped volume will vary form one area of the lung to another. (3) The auto-PEEP, as measured on a manometer, is an average of the pressure level throughout the lung. (4) The auto-PEEP reading on the manometer underestimates the actual mean auto-PEEP in the lungs. During active exhalation the ventilator manometer often reads zero or the set PEEP level but not auto-PEEP. This indicates that the pressure in the circuit is zero or the set PEEP level. When checking for auto-PEEP, at the end of exhalation when the expiratory valve is occluded but the patient does not receive an inspiration, the manometer will increase its reading if auto-PEEP is present. Since the "extra pressure" in the lung (auto-PEEP) must repressurize the circuit, the final pressure recorded is actually less than the real auto-PEEP level. (5) Auto-PEEP will increase the work of breathing for a patient who is breathing spontaneously while on a mechanical ventilator. To create a negative pressure or inspiratory flow great enough to allow the ventilator to sense the effort, the patient must overcome the effects of the increased positive pressure (auto-PEEP) in his lungs. The machine cannot compensate for this, and the situation is analogous to decreasing the sensitivity setting on a patient without auto-PEEP.

Ventilation Exercises

For each of the following calculations, use the equations from Respiratory Care, *Chapter 12, Equation Box 2.*

12-11. Given:

PIP = 40 cmH$_2$O	PEEP = 8 cmH$_2$O
T$_I$ = 0.8 sec	f = 20 breaths/min
set V$_T$ = 800 mL	Insp flow = 60 L/min
Pplat = 27 cmH$_2$O	Peak exp flow = 40 L/min
Cf = 2 mL/cmH$_2$O	auto-PEEP = 3 cmH$_2$O

Calculate:

mean Paw (const pres vent)	_____	cmH$_2$O
mean Paw (const vol vent)	_____	cmH$_2$O
Corrected V$_T$	_____	mL
Compliance (V$_T$ corrected)	_____	mL/cmH$_2$O
Compliance (V$_T$ not corrected)	_____	mL/cmH$_2$O
R$_I$	_____	cmH$_2$O/L/sec
R$_E$	_____	cmH$_2$O/L/sec
W	_____	kg-M

12-12. Given:

PIP = 22 cmH$_2$O	PEEP = 5 cmH$_2$O
T$_I$ = 1.2 sec	f = 10 breaths/min
set V$_T$ = 600 mL	Insp flow = 30 L/min
Pplat = 18 cmH$_2$O	Peak exp flow = 20 L/min
Cf = 2 mL/cmH$_2$O	auto-PEEP = 0 cmH$_2$O

Calculate:

mean Paw (const pres vent)	_____	cmH$_2$O
mean Paw (const vol vent)	_____	cmH$_2$O
Corrected V$_T$	_____	mL
Compliance (V$_T$ corrected)	_____	mL/cmH$_2$O
Compliance (V$_T$ not corrected)	_____	mL/cmH$_2$O
R$_I$	_____	cmH$_2$O/L/sec
R$_E$	_____	cmH$_2$O/L/sec
W	_____	kg-M

Invasive Monitoring Calculations

For each of the following calculations, refer to Respiratory Care, *Chapter 12, Equation Box 5. For review of oxygen content formulas, refer to Chapter 9 in this book.*

12-13. Given:

PaO$_2$ = 90 mmHg	SaO$_2$ = 96% (0.96)
COHb = 1% (0.01)	(corrected for CO and
FiO$_2$ = 40% (0.40)	Met Hb)
PvO$_2$ = 35 mmHg	metHb = 1% (0.01)
EBP = 713 mmHg	PaCO$_2$ = 48 mmHg
	SvO$_2$ (HbO$_2$) = 69% (0.69)
	Hb = 14 g/dL

Calculate:

P$_A$O$_2$	_____	mmHg
Sc'O$_2$	_____	%
Cc'O$_2$	_____	mL oxygen/dL blood
CaO$_2$	_____	mL oxygen/dL blood
CvO$_2$	_____	mL oxygen/dL blood
Qs/Qt	_____	% (using the shunt equation)

12-14. Given:

PaO$_2$ = 200 mmHg	FiO$_2$ = 80% (0.80)
PaCO$_2$ = 36 mmHg	P$_A$O$_2$ = 400 mmHg

Calculate:

Qs/Qt _____ % (using the modified shunt equation)

Physiologic Dead Space Exercises

For each of the following calculations, refer to Respiratory Care, *Chapter 12, Equation Box #6.*

12-15. Given:

PaCO$_2$ = 40 mmHg	P$_E$CO$_2$ = 27 mmHg
V$_T$ = 600 mL	

Calculate:

V$_D$/V$_T$	_____	
V$_D$	_____	mL

12-16. Given:

PaCO$_2$ = 40 mmHg	P$_E$CO$_2$ = 20 mmHg
V$_T$ = 400 mL	

Calculate:

V$_D$/V$_T$	_____	
V$_D$	_____	mL

12-17. Given:

PaCO$_2$ = 60 mmHg	P$_E$CO$_2$ = 36 mmHg
V$_T$ = 700 mL	

Calculate:

V$_D$/V$_T$	_____	
V$_D$	_____	mL

Capnography Exercises

12-18. Identify and explain each of the following points and segments found in the following tracing.

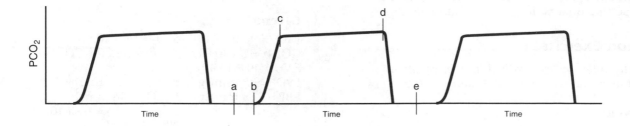

a. point a: _____
b. segment a-b: _____
c. segment b-c: _____
d. segment c-d: _____
e. point d: _____
f. segment d-e: _____
g. point e: _____

REVIEW QUESTIONS

12-19. Which of the following would decrease afterload?
A. dopamine
B. phenylephrine
C. nitroglycerine
D. norepinephrine

12-20. With normal $\dot{V}/\dot{Q}$, the $P_{ET}CO_2$ will most closely approximate which of the following?
A. P_vCO_2
B. P_aCO_2
C. P_ICO_2
D. P_ACO_2

12-21. Which of the following is not correct concerning transcutaneous monitoring?
A. $P_{tc}O_2$ is often lower than P_aO_2
B. $P_{tc}CO_2$ is often higher than P_aCO_2
C. $P_{tc}CO_2$ decreases with decreased perfusion
D. the $P_{tc}O_2$ monitor must be heated to approximate P_aO_2

12-22. The major advantage of the closed-circuit over the open-circuit indirect calorimetry method is:
A. ability to measure V_T
B. ability to make measurements at a high F_IO_2
C. the ability to disregard leaks
D. the shorter time required for testing

12-23. Each of the following is true concerning monitoring except:
A. it may be invasive or noninvasive
B. it may be continuous or intermittent
C. it results in delayed-time assessment
D. it results in little or no blood loss from the patient

12-24. Hazards of pulse oximeter use include all of the following except:
A. burns
B. bleeding
C. pressure necrosis
D. inaccuracy with fetal hemoglobin

12-25. Each of the following may affect the accuracy of pulse oximeters except:
A. carboxyhemoglobin (COHb)
B. methylene blue dye
C. vascular infusion of lipids
D. deeply pigmented skin

12-26. A pressure-volume curve is recorded for a patient on mechanical ventilation. Two hours later, the patient has increased airway resistance, but his compliance has not changed. Which of the following is correct?
A. the pressure-volume curve would be wider
B. the pressure-volume curve would be skinnier
C. the slope of the pressure-volume curve would be more vertical
D. the slope of the pressure-volume curve would be more horizontal

12-27. A pressure-volume curve is recorded for a patient on mechanical ventilation. Two hours later, the patient has decreased compliance, but his airway resistance has not changed. Which of the following is correct?
A. the pressure-volume curve would be wider
B. the pressure-volume curve would be skinnier
C. the slope of the pressure-volume curve would be more vertical
D. the slope of the pressure-volume curve would be more horizontal

SECTION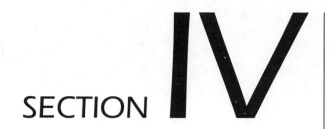

RESPIRATORY CARE MODALITIES AND EQUIPMENT

13

Medical Gas Therapy

Oxygen is a drug, a fact that is often overlooked because of its routine use. The delivery of medical gases (especially oxygen) to patients is accomplished through the use of various types of respiratory therapy equipment. This chapter discusses air compressors, oxygen concentrators, liquid oxygen systems, gas cylinders, the use of pressure-reducing devices (regulators), flow-controlling devices (flowmeters), and oxygen therapy devices that are responsible for providing an oxygen-enriched environment. The effect oxygen administration has on the alveolar and arterial partial pressure of oxygen is also discussed.

AIR COMPRESSORS

Compressed air can be supplied from tanks but is more frequently supplied by electrical compressors. In the hospital setting, the compressor can be a bedside device or air can be piped into the patient's room from a large compressor elsewhere. Compressors are one of three types: diaphragm, piston, or rotary. The small, portable-type compressors used to deliver low flows or pressures are usually diaphragm compressors. Piston compressors are routinely used when high flows or pressures are required. Compressed air can be used for the delivery of aerosols, to power intermittent positive pressure breathing (IPPB) machines or mechanical ventilators, and to supply air to air/oxygen blenders, power tents, and so forth. Two of the main hazards associated with the use of portable machines are electrical safety and overheating of the compressor.

Exercise 1

Obtain two air compressors, one large and one small, and perform the following exercises:

13-1. Using a manometer, check the maximum operating pressure of the compressor. Is it adjustable?

13-2. Using a flow measuring device, document the maximum flow rates obtainable from the compressor. Is there a relationship between flow rate and operating pressure?

13-3. Identify the alarms found on the compressors. Create an alarm situation and check to see if the alarm is functional.

OXYGEN CONCENTRATORS

Oxygen concentrators have the ability to separate oxygen from the other gases in the atmosphere and deliver it to patients in concentrations of greater than 21%. The molecular sieve-type concentrator delivers high concentrations of oxygen, 86% to 97%, depending on the flow rate used. The permeable membrane or enricher-type concentrator delivers approximately 40% oxygen at various flow rates.

Exercise 2

Obtain a molecular sieve oxygen concentrator and perform the following exercises:

13-4. Document the percent oxygen delivery by analyzing the gas coming from the device at different flow rates.

13-5. Using a manometer, check the operating pressure of the system by connecting it to the outlet port of the unit.

13-6. Using a flow measuring device, document accurate flow rates by measuring the flow delivered by the unit.

GAS CYLINDERS

Gas cylinders used in a hospital setting are usually made from heat-treated steel. These cylinders (or tanks) are discussed in this section. Although the actual pressures and resultant number of liters of gas for a given cylinder size may vary slightly from manufacturer to manufacturer, the values that will be used for the discussion of oxygen cylinders are listed in Table 13-1. I would recommend memorizing these values for full cylinders. The volume of a full cylinder can be expressed in cubic feet, gallons, liters (L) or any other volume expression. Since liters are the most com-

TABLE 13-1 **Common Cylinder Sizes Along With Their Filling Volumes, Pressures for Full Cylinders, and the Cylinder Factors**

Cylinder Size	Liters (L)	Pressure (psig)	Factor (L/psig)
D	360	2200	0.16
E	620	2200	0.28
M	3000	2200	1.36
G	5300	2200	2.41
H	6900	2200	3.14

monly used form of expression, especially when it comes to oxygen delivery to patients, it is probably best to memorize the liter values.

Because tanks have a relatively small, limited volume of gas available for use, the user should know how to calculate the length of time a cylinder will deliver the appropriate flow of oxygen. The volumes for full gaseous cylinders are already listed, but there are two ways to determine the actual volume of partially filled cylinders. One is by using the cylinder factor, the other is by setting up a mathematical relationship. (Liquid tanks must be weighed and are not discussed here.) The cylinder factor is considered first. This factor is determined by dividing the volume of a full tank by the pressure of a full tank.

Example: Determination of the Cylinder Factor

A full "E" cylinder contains 620 L at a pressure of 2200 psig.

$$620 \text{ L}/2200 \text{ psig} = 0.28 \text{ L/psig.}$$

For every 1 psig generated, there will be 0.28 L of gas in the tank. This value is relatively constant from 0 to 2200 psig and can be used to determine tank contents in liters at any pressure.

Example: Determination of Tank Contents Using The Cylinder Factor

An "E" cylinder at 2200 psig will contain 620 L of oxygen.

$$2200 \times 0.28 = 620 \text{ (a full cylinder)}$$

An "E" cylinder at 1000 psig will contain 280 L of oxygen.

$$1000 \times 0.28 = 280$$
(this cylinder is less than half full)

If a practitioner does not want to memorize the cylinder factors, or to calculate them each time a volume determination must be made, the second method using the following mathematical relationship can be used:

$$\frac{\text{volume of full cylinder}}{\text{pressure of full cylinder}} = \frac{\text{volume of partially full cylinder}}{\text{pressure of a partially full cylinder}}$$

Example

An "E" cylinder has a pressure of 1000 psig. How many liters are present?

$$\frac{620 \text{ L}}{2200 \text{ psig}} = \frac{X}{1000 \text{ psig}} \quad X = 282 \text{ L}$$

When comparing the two methods (check the two examples above, 280 L compared with 282 L), a slightly different value may result since the value of 0.28 and the other tank factors are rounded off. This process will work for any size gaseous tank. (Not tanks with liquid in them.)

Once the cylinder contents are known, the duration of time it may be used can be calculated if the flow rate being used is also known. The "E" cylinder, in the previous example, contains 280 L. If oxygen is being used at 4 L/min the cylinder will last for 70 minutes (280 L/4 L/min = 70 minutes). Obviously, a full tank should be on standby for use when the one being used runs low. All respiratory care departments should have a protocol for changing cylinders. Often cylinders will be taken out of service when their pressure drops below 500 psig.

Cylinder Contents and Time of Use Calculations

For each of the following situations, determine the volume of oxygen contained in the cylinder and the maximum time period for which it can be used. (You may wish to compare both methods for determining the cylinder contents.)

	Cylinder Size	psig	Liter Flow	Cylinder Volume	Time Period
13-7.	E	50	4 L/min	____	____
13-8.	E	1200	10 L/min	____	____
13-9.	D	500	5 L/min	____	____
13-10.	D	1800	2 L/min	____	____
13-11.	H	800	6 L/min	____	____
13-12.	H	1500	3 L/min	____	____

Tank Pressure Calculations

Using the same formulas, calculate the pressure in the following cylinders if the volume is known. This is purely an academic exercise. Clinically you cannot know the actual number of liters until you calculate them based on the pressure.

	Cylinder Size	Liters	Cylinder Pressure
13-13.	G	1200	____
13-14.	H (K)	4000	____
13-15.	M (F)	900	____
13-16.	D	80	____
13-17.	E	250	____

Clinical Problem-Solving

13-18. How many "G" cylinders would it take to supply the oxygen needed for continuous use to a home patient who is receiving 4 L/min for 1 full week?

13-19. How long will a full "E" cylinder last during the transport of a patient on a portable mechanical ventilator where the ventilator is set at a tidal volume of 800 mL, the actual frequency is 14 breaths/min, and 5 L/min is also being used by the ventilator to allow it to perform its functions?

Exercise 3

13-20. *Obtain several gas cylinders of different sizes and gas contents and perform the following:*
   a. Compare the color codes for the different gases.
   b. Identify the markings on the cylinders.
   c. Read the label attached to the cylinder.
   d. Safely transport both a small and large cylinder using the appropriate transport carts.

   e. Compare the design of the tank valve outlets on both a small and large cylinder. What safety systems are present and how do they differ for different gases?
   f. Locate the pressure-release devices on both small and large cylinders.

13-21. "Crack" a cylinder by slowly opening the cylinder valve. Why is this done?

LIQUID OXYGEN

Liquid oxygen changes to gaseous oxygen when it reaches its boiling point. At one atmospheric pressure (Patm), this occurs at approximately −183°C. This phenomenon of liquid turning to gas takes place in both large bulk oxygen delivery systems for hospitals and in small portable systems for individual patient use. The actual temperature at which this change occurs varies depending on the pressure in the system. One cubic foot equals 28.3 L (this applies to gas or liquid volume). One liter of liquid oxygen weighs 2.5 lb, and 1 L of liquid oxygen will "evaporate" to become 860 L of gaseous oxygen.

Clinical Problem-Solving

Using the above information, calculate the following:

13-22. Two pounds of liquid oxygen in a portable unit will last what maximum time if a patient is using a continuous flow of 4 L/min?

13-23. How many pounds of liquid oxygen will be used in a week by a home patient using 5 L/min continuously?

13-24. How many "E" cylinders would be needed to equal the gas volume of a hospital's liquid system, which contains 50 cubic feet of liquid oxygen?

Exercise 4

Obtain a liquid oxygen reservoir system for home use and perform the following exercises:

13-25. Document the percent oxygen delivery by analyzing the gas coming from the device.

13-26. Using a manometer, check the operating pressure of the system by connecting it to the outlet port of the unit.

13-27. Using a flow-measuring device, document accurate flow rates by measuring the flow delivered by the unit.

13-28. Determine the fullness of the tank. Is it based on a pressure reading?

13-29. Practice filling a portable unit from the stationary liquid tank.

13-30. Locate the liquid oxygen tank at your institution and identify the following: the liquid storage tank, the vaporizer coils, the backup system, and the indicator gauges. Is its location appropriate in relation to nearby structures? Locate the area inside the institution where the pipes enter. Identify the main delivery pipe, the main shut-off valve, and some zone valves located throughout the institution.

13-31. Using a Bourdon pressure gauge, measure the pressure in the oxygen and air lines delivering pressure to a station outlet.

13-32. Consider touring a liquid oxygen processing plant.

SAFETY SYSTEMS

There are two safety systems associated with gas cylinder outlets and regulator inlets, The American Standard Safety System (ASSS), formerly known as the thread index safety system (TISS), and the Pin Index Safety System (PISS). ASSS connectors allow joining of a regulator with large cylinders (M, G, and H). These connectors are threaded adapters that are manufactured so that only appropriate regulators and cylinders can be matched. PISS connectors allow joining of a regulator with a small cylinder (A through E). The PISS is comprised of two holes in the neck of the cylinder and two pins on the yoke of the regulator. Pin and hole placement only allow appropriate matches between regulators and cylinders. If the pins are removed, the safety of the system is voided. Another safety system, the Diameter Index Safety System (DISS), is also a threaded system similar to the ASSS, but it is used where pressures are less than 200 psig (connectors distal to the reducing valve). This adapter allows connection between flowmeters and other respiratory therapy equipment. Two of the most commonly used type of connectors are for air and oxygen, each having a separate DISS designation. Although flowmeters are available with appropriate air and oxygen DISS adapters, many air flowmeters are manufactured with an oxygen DISS adapter. This allows interchanging of equipment between flowmeters and saves time, money, and equipment storage space. However, this practice increases the chance of delivering an incorrect gas. Extra care must be taken to make sure the appropriate gas is being used. It is also important to note that not all threaded connectors are part of the safety systems described. The "permanent" connectors are pipe threads. They are not routinely unthreaded from their connectors.

REGULATORS

The typical regulator encountered in routine use is found connected to a gas cylinder. Regulators have three basic components that perform three functions. Regulators have a pressure-reducing valve or chamber for reducing pressures to an appropriate level. They have gauges for measuring cylinder contents. They also have a flow regulating/measuring device for controlling the flow of gas to be used. Regulators may be classified as direct-acting or indirect-acting, single-stage, or multi-stage, and as adjustable or nonadjustable (preset). The terms "adjustable" and "preset" refer to the method of operation of the device. Adjustable regulators allow change of flow to occur through the adjustment of pressure. Preset regulators are routinely set for a 50 psig outlet pressure, and flow is adjusted by means of a flow-regulating device (Thorpe tube). They need to be checked for proper operation periodically and adjusted as needed to maintain outlet pressure at 50 psig.

Since most regulators are found attached to cylinders, it is important to understand the proper method to attach and remove regulators. Before attaching a regulator, the cylinder should be "cracked." This means the cylinder valve should be opened, and some gas should be allowed to escape. This will remove any dirt or debris in the cylinder outlet port, and also document that the cylinder is pressurized.

Regulators with ASSS connectors can be threaded directly onto the cylinder. A large wrench is needed to tighten the adapter. Regulators with PISS adapters need a small plastic O-ring to create a seal between the regulator and the cylinder valve outlet so there is no leak. The yoke may be tightened by hand or with a small tool. Once the regulator is firmly in place, the tank valve should be pressurized slowly. If a leak is detected, close the tank valve and recheck connectors. Before removing a regulator, the needle valve on the tank must be closed and the regulator depressurized.

FLOWMETERS

Devices that regulate and measure flow are commonly referred to as flowmeters. Flowmeters operate on the principle of a fixed or variable orifice. They are powered by a fixed or variable pressure. This results in a fixed or variable flow.

Flow Restrictors

Flow restrictors work off of a fixed pressure, have a fixed orifice, and deliver a fixed flow rate. Flow restrictors will only be accurate if the driving pressure remains constant at the pressure for which they were calibrated, the orifice is unobstructed, minimal back pressure from downstream resistance is encountered, and they are used with the intended gas.

Bourdon Gauges

Bourdon gauges work off of a variable pressure, have a fixed orifice, and can deliver a variable flow rate. Bourdon gauges measure pressure. Those used to measure tank contents are calibrated in pressure units. Those used to indicate flow are calibrated in flow units. Bourdon gauges used to indicate flow will deliver less gas than indicated in the face of back pressure. They will, however, read accurately in any position, and this makes them desirable for use when cylinders must be moved around and placed on their side.

Thorpe Tubes

Thorpe tubes work off of a fixed pressure, have a variable orifice, and can deliver a variable flow rate. Thorpe tubes can be divided into two general categories, back pressure compensated, and non–back pressure compensated. Actual flow will be higher than indicated flow in the face of back pressure with non–back pressure compensated Thorpe tubes. Consequently, they are not and should not be used in clinical practice.

Thorpe tubes are calibrated to deliver accurate flow when operating at 760 mmHg (1 Patm), 70°F, and 50 psig internal pressure. Because of this, Thorpe tubes should never be used in combination with an adjustable regulator. Flowmeters are also calibrated for the density of the gas for which they are to be used. Inaccurate flows will result if gases of different densities from those for which the flowmeter is intended are delivered through a flowmeter of any type. Decreased density will result in increased flows; increased density will result in decreased flows.

Although Thorpe tubes must be upright to read the flow accurately, once the flow is set, placing a Thorpe tube on its side will not result in a change of flow. The needle valve controls the flow, not the ball. The ball only indicates the flow.

Thorpe tubes may come calibrated for different levels of flow: 0 to 1 L/min, 0 to 3 L/min, 0 to 15 L/min, or 0 to 75 L/min. Although they are calibrated for accurate flow, flows greater than the calibrated scale are possible as long as the outlet flow does not encounter excessive back pressure. Many Thorpe-type flowmeters set in the "flush" region will allow over 100 L/min unrestricted flow to exit from them when the needle valve is opened fully.

Exercise 5

13-33. Examine a large cylinder's ASSS and its associated regulator. Practice connecting and disconnecting the regulator.

13-34. Examine a small cylinder's PISS and its associated regulator. Practice connecting and disconnecting the regulator.

13-35. Examine both the air and oxygen DISS connectors. How are they different? Where can you find actual air DISS connectors?

13-36. Compare the pressure release valve (pop-off) on a regulator with that on a gas cylinder.

13-37. Obtain both a pressure preset and pressure adjustable regulator. Compare the two regulators.

13-38. Disassemble and correctly reassemble a regulator identifying the following: gas inlet, gas outlet, pressure chamber, ambient chamber, diaphragm, spring, pressure gauge, and pressure release. Is it a direct-acting or indirect-acting pressure regulator?

13-39. Obtain the following flow measuring/regulating devices: Bourdon gauge, Thorpe tube, and flow restrictor. Compare them, classifying each as a fixed orifice/variable orifice, fixed pressure/variable pressure, and fixed flow/variable flow device.

13-40. Attach an adjustable regulator with a Bourdon gauge to a gas cylinder. Set the flow at 6 L/min. Completely occlude the outlet and observe the flow indicator.

13-41. Test a Thorpe tube flowmeter for back pressure compensation by performing one or more of the following: (Comments refer to compensated flow tubes)
  1. Read the label. (It is written there.)
  2. With the needle valve closed, plug it into a 50 psig gas source. (The ball will jump.)
  3. Measure the flow in the face of back pressure. (The flow will drop as back pressure is increased but the flow will be accurate.)
  4. Determine the placement of the needle valve. (Placed after the flow tube.)

13-42. Obtain both back pressure and non–back pressure compensated Thorpe tubes. Connect them to a 50 psig gas source. Set the flow at 10 L/min and measure it. If it is accurate, it should be delivering 10 L/min. Apply back pressure to the flowmeters. What happens to the set flow compared with the actual flow with the pressure compensated tube? The non–back pressure compensated tube?

13-43. Obtain a back pressure compensated Thorpe tube and connect it to an adjustable regulator. (**This should never be done in clinical practice.**) Using a pressure gauge, set the regulator at 20 psig outlet pressure. Adjust the flow on the flowmeter to 10 L/min. Measure the actual flow. How do they compare? Repeat this at 30, 40, 50, 60, 70, and 80 psig. Always reset the flow at 10 L/min before measuring the actual flow rate.

13-44. Attach a preset regulator with a Thorpe tube to an E cylinder. Set the flow at 6 L/min and measure it. Now place the E cylinder on its side and continue to measure the actual flow. What happens to the flow indicator? Does actual flow change?

13-45. Obtain a flow-measuring device capable of measuring continuous flow at over 100 L/min. Place a Thorpe tube into a 50 psig wall outlet and slowly open the needle valve the whole way. Document the flow output.

OXYGEN THERAPY DEVICES

Oxygen therapy devices can be classified into two groups: low-flow, variable performance devices, or high-flow, fixed performance devices. The use of low-flow devices will result in a variable FiO_2 as the patient's respiratory rate, VT, I:E ratio, and so forth, change. In some cases, FiO_2 will vary with mouth or nose breathing. The use of high-flow devices will result in a constant FiO_2 regardless of the patient's breathing pattern. This is because high-flow devices are intended to meet or exceed the patient's inspiratory demand. High-flow devices include air-entrainment masks (AEMs), large volume aerosol systems, large-volume humidifier systems, oxygen hoods, isolettes (incubators), and tents. Mechanical ventilators and intermittent mandatory ventilation (IMV) and continuous positive airway pressure (CPAP) systems would also fit into this category. Low-flow devices include nasal catheters, nasal cannulas, transtracheal catheters, simple masks, partial rebreathing masks (PRMs), and non-rebreathing masks (NRMs).

Summary of Common Devices

The various types of oxygen therapy devices are explained in the text. Following is a brief summary.

Nasal catheter: Rarely used.

Nasal cannula: Commonly used because of ease of use and good tolerance by patients. However, delivered FiO_2 is difficult, if not impossible, to calculate or even estimate. It is the second best choice of the oxygen therapy devices for patients with chronic obstructive pulmonary disease (COPD) in acute exacerbations or in unstable conditions. Remember that cannulas are only useful if the patient has patent nasal passages.

Simple masks: These devices should be last in line when considering the choices of oxygen therapy equipment. Low flows may result in rebreathing of CO_2 and heat buildup in the mask. If low FiO_2s are desired, an AEM should be used. If high FiO_2s are desired, a PRM or NRM should be used. A simple mask should be used when other oxygen equipment is unavailable. Some simple masks are manufactured with the small-bore oxygen tubing adapter made to entrain room air. This increases the total flow into the mask and helps maintain a more constant FiO_2.

Partial rebreathing and non-rebreathing masks: PRMs and NRMs can deliver relatively high FiO_2s when using high flow rates and a tight-fitting mask. The premise that the first third of a patient's exhaled gas enters the reservoir bag when using a PRM needs further investigation. In some situations, the patient's exhaled gas will most likely take the path of least resistance, which is between a loosely fitting mask and the patient's face or through the exhalation valves with little gas entering the reservoir bag. The oxygen flow rate into the bag, the actual bag distention, and the patient's exhaled volume and flow rate also likely play a role in this matter.

Air-entrainment masks: AEMs should be the oxygen delivery device of choice when a known FiO_2 is desired. They should be the first choice for patients with unstable COPD. After the acute exacerbation has passed, they may be exchanged for a cannula. For entrainment devices, the size of the jet and the size of the entrainment ports (windows) control the air:O_2 ratio, thus the FiO_2. Small jets result in increased room air entrainment and lower FiO_2s. Small ports allow less entrainment and increased FiO_2s. The source gas flow influences total gas flow, but changes in source gas flow should not change the air:O_2 ratio, and thus have minimal effects on the FiO_2.

Oxygen hoods: These are used for treatment of neonates. They produce a controlled environment of temperature, humidity, and FiO_2. The flow of oxygen delivered by an oxygen hood should always be warmed and humidified. Temperature and FiO_2 should be constantly monitored. Suggested flows vary from a minimum of 7 L/min recommended for small hoods to 10 to 12 L/min minimum for large hoods. This flow should help guarantee that an appropriate FiO_2 will be maintained, and that carbon dioxide will be washed out of the hood. Oxygen hoods can be used independently or in conjunction with an isolette (incubator).

Tents: Tent therapy is most often used for older infants and pediatric patients. Goals of tent therapy include: maintaining a constant FiO_2, maintaining a subambient temperature, delivery of humidity, and providing an isolated environment. Although often referred to as "O_2 tents," compressed air can be used to power the tent if oxygen concentrations greater than 21% are not required. The FiO_2 in a tent will vary depending on the delivered FiO_2, the total flow into the tent, the tent canopy volume, how tightly the canopy fits the bed, and how often the canopy is opened and closed. Total flow into the tent (greater than 15 L/min) should be high enough to provide a constant FiO_2, and to wash out the CO_2 exhaled by the patient. FiO_2s may vary from 0.21 to 0.50. Environmental temperature can be influenced by evaporative cooling (very inefficient), the use of ice, or by the use of a refrigeration unit. This temperature will vary depending on the efficiency of the cooling unit, the size of the canopy, how well the canopy fits the bed, how often the canopy is opened, the room temperature, and possibly the patient's size and body temperature. Because a cool environment is usually desired during tent therapy, its use is not indicated for newborns who require a warm environment. Humidity is delivered in the form of an aerosol via an atomizer or some type of nebulizer.

The term "croup tent" is also widely used because tents are a common method of treatment for patients with croup. Tents are also used for special purposes such as Ribavirin therapy for patients with bronchiolitis. Some of the hazards of tent therapy include the following: development of bronchospasms from the inhaled water particles, infection due to contaminated aerosols, difficulty of patient inspection in a dense aerosol, and a fire hazard with the increased oxygen environment. Electrical or spark-generating devices should not be allowed in or near a tent.

Exercise 6

13-46. Obtain each of the following: a nasal cannula, an AEM, and an NRM. Appropriately place each of these devices on a mannequin or classmate at the proper flow.

13-47. Obtain a 40% AEM:
1. Set it up with the source gas flow at 10 L/min and analyze the FIO_2.
2. Turn the source gas flow to 8 L/min and 12 L/min and re-analyze at each setting. What happens to the FIO_2?
3. Block the entrainment ports and re-measure the FIO_2. What happens to the FIO_2?

GAS MIXING

Gas mixing allows the clinician to deliver precise O_2 concentrations to patients by mixing varying amounts of air and O_2. The use of a blender is an easy way to mix two gases. Routinely, the two gases are air and oxygen, although others such as nitric oxide or helium may be used in the clinical setting. The two source gases both at approximately 50 psig enter the blender. Through a process of pressure adjustment and blending, the two gases are mixed to an appropriate FIO_2. The gas leaves the device via a flow meter or other flow-controlling device. Concentrations of 21% to 100% oxygen are available and easily adjustable with these devices. Blenders are often incorporated into mechanical ventilators for ease of adjusting FIO_2. They are also used as free-standing devices for oxygen delivery. Another method for mixing gases is to use two flowmeters, one connected to compressed air and the other oxygen. The flows from each of these devices would then be mixed together for an appropriate FIO_2. A calculation of FIO_2 can be done when mixing any proportions of air and O_2 by using the following formula.

$$V1 \times C1 + V2 \times C2 = Vt \times Ct$$

Where:

V1 is the volume of room air
C1 is the FO_2 in room air (0.21)
V2 is the volume of O_2
C2 is the FO_2 of 100% O_2 (1.0)
Vt is the total volume of the mixture
Ct is the final concentration of the mixture

Example

7 L of air is mixed with 3 L of O_2

$$7 \times 0.21 + 3 \times 1 = 10 \times Ct$$

$$(1.47 + 3)/10 = Ct$$

$$Ct = 0.447 \text{ or } 45\% \text{ } O_2$$

Oxygen Percent Calculations

Calculate the percent O_2 that results from mixing the following amounts of air and O_2.

	Mixtures	O_2 Percent (%)
13-48.	18 L of air and 18 L of O_2	_____
13-49.	4 L of air and 4 L of O_2	_____
13-50.	15 L of air and 4 L of O_2	_____
13-51.	6 L of air and 14 L of O_2	_____
13-52.	19 L of air and 34 L of O_2	_____

Please notice from 13-48 and 13-49 that it is the ratio of air to oxygen that is mixed that determines the resultant FIO_2 and not the total amount of gas that is mixed together. This concept is important in the next discussion on entrainment.

GAS ENTRAINMENT

Entrainment provides another method of mixing gases. Gas entrainment devices are routinely powered by 100% oxygen and room air that is entrained. Entrainment (or jet mixing) devices "entrain" room air at a preset ratio determined by the size of the entrainment port (or window) and the size of the jet. Since the ratio of air to oxygen remains constant, once set, the FIO_2 delivered by these devices remains rather constant even if the flow rate set on the flow meter is changed. To determine the ratio for any given FO_2, the V1C1 formula can be used or the "X method" can be used.

Example: V1C1 Formula

Determine the ratio of air to O_2 (A:O_2) for 40% O_2.

$$V1 \times C1 + V2 \times C2 = Vt \times Ct$$

To determine ratios, always allow V2 (the volume of O_2) to equal 1.

$$Z \times 0.21 + 1 \times 1 = (Z + 1) \times 0.4$$
$$0.21Z + 1 = 0.4Z + 0.4{:}0.6 = 0.19Z{:}Z = 3.16$$

The A:O_2 ratio for 40% O_2 is approximately 3:1.

Example: The "X Method"

Determine the A:O_2 ratio for 40% O_2 by using the "X method" (Figure 13-1).

1. Place the desired O_2 percent in the middle of the X.
2. Place 21 (21% O_2) in the left upper arm of the X.
3. Place 100 (100% O_2) in the left lower leg of the X.

4. Now, following the X pattern, subtract, placing the differences in the right-sided arm and leg. (Keep all numbers positive.)
5. Divide the value in the right lower leg into both the right upper arm and the right lower leg. This always makes the O_2 value = 1.
6. The result of the right upper arm:right lower leg ratio is the A:O_2 ratio for the O_2% in the middle of the X.

Either method is accurate for determining the A:O_2 ratio for any FO_2, although rounding off (eg, room air = 21%), regardless of the method used, can make the numbers slightly inaccurate. Some of the common ratios are listed in Table 13-2.

TABLE 13-2   **A:O_2 Ratios for Common FIO_2s**

A	O_2	Actual O_2%	Commonly Stated O_2%
0.6	1	70.4	70
1.0	1	60.5	60
2.0	1	47.3	47
3.0	1	40.7	40
4.0	1	36.8	37
5.0	1	34.2	35
10.0	1	28.2	28
25.0	1	24.0	24

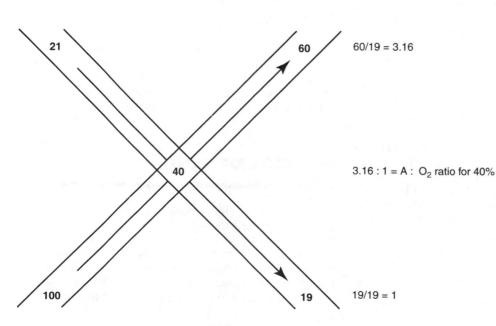

60/19 = 3.16

3.16 : 1 = A : O_2 ratio for 40%

19/19 = 1

FIGURE 13-1. The X method.

Air:Oxygen Ratio Calculations

Calculate the ratios for the following FIO_2s. Try using both methods. For consistency, always make $O_2 = 1$ in the ratio.

	O₂ Percent	V1C1 Formula A:O₂	X Method A:O₂
13-53.	24%	_____	_____
13-54.	26%	_____	_____
13-55.	32%	_____	_____
13-56.	45%	_____	_____
13-57.	65%	_____	_____
13-58.	85%	_____	_____

TOTAL FLOW OUTPUT

When working with nebulizers and other entrainment devices, another important consideration is the total flow output of the device. Entrainment devices are classified as high-flow systems, and should therefore provide enough flow output to meet or exceed the inspiratory flow rates of the patient. The purpose for meeting the patient's inspiratory demands is to make sure that the patient is receiving the appropriate FIO_2 as delivered by the device. If the flow rate delivered from the device is too low, the patient will inhale room air along with the FIO_2 delivered by the device, thus diluting the delivered FIO_2.

Routinely patients receiving O_2 from a high-flow system do not have their inspiratory flow rate (FR), inspiratory time (TI), or tidal volume (VT) measured. If resting peak inspiratory flow rate was known, the output from the system could be set to match it. If TI and VT were known, the average inspiratory flow rate could be calculated by the following formula:

$$FR \text{ (L/min)} = VT \text{ (L)} \times 60 \text{ (sec/min)}/TI \text{ (sec)}$$

Knowing these parameters would help guide the use of appropriate flow output from the entrainment device. Since FR, TI, and VT are not routinely known, practitioners guess at the appropriate flow rates. A flow of 30 to 40 L/min would be a recommended *minimum* for these devices when used with adults. For many patients, a flow of 60 L/min or greater would be more appropriate. If an aerosol is being delivered, the necessary flow rate can be estimated by observing the patient during inspiration. If the aerosol exiting the mask or T-piece "disappears" from the exhalation port during inspiration, the flow from the device may need to be increased.

Calculation of Total Flow Output

The total flow rate (FRt) delivered from an entrainment device can be calculated by knowing the source gas flow rate (FRsg, the O_2 flow meter setting) and the ratio of air to oxygen for the delivered FIO_2. For a given FIO_2, add the ratio value for air (A), to the ratio value for O_2 (which is always 1), and then multiply that value by the flowmeter setting. This relationship is expressed in the following formula:

$$FRt = FRsg \text{ (A + O2 ratio values)}$$

Example

40% O_2 is being delivered with a flow meter set at 8 L/min. What is the total flow being delivered to the patient? The A:O_2 ratio is 3:1

$$FRt = 8 (3 + 1) = 8 \times 4 = 32 \text{ L/min}$$

Total Flow Calculations: Student Exercise

Calculate the total flow from entrainment devices under the following conditions:

	FIO₂ Setting (%)	Flow Setting (L/min)	Total Flow (L/min)
13-59.	40	10	_____
13-60.	37	9	_____
13-61.	34	8	_____
13-62.	28	5	_____
13-63.	24	4	_____
13-64.	47	13	_____
13-65.	55	15	_____
13-66.	75	15	_____

I would like to address two problems encountered when using nebulizers for FIO_2 and aerosol delivery. The first is difficulty in delivering high FIO_2s at a high total gas flow. This occurs because the jets in many entrainment devices are very small. Their size allows appropriate entrainment for the given port size but it limits the amount of flow through the jet at 50 psi driving pressure. Thus, with high FIO_2 settings, total flow is lower than the patients inspiratory flow rate. Room air is often inhaled thus diluting the delivered FIO_2 by the device. To help correct the problem, two devices must be connected together so total flow can be increased. Even this is not sufficient sometimes. Make sure the final output is analyzed, in that back pressure may affect the entrainment of the devices. Another option is to use a device manufactured specifically for high flows at increased FIO_2s.

A second problem is encountered at low FIO_2s. Some nebulizers when set at a low FIO_2, deliver such a poor aerosol density (mg water/L gas) that it can be questioned whether the humidity therapy is of any benefit. One way to combat this problem is to use a blender in conjunction with a nebulizer. The problem can be addressed by placing the nebulizer on an entrainment setting, which delivers a good aerosol density, and then placing the blender setting at an FIO_2 lower than 100% oxygen to achieve the desired FIO_2 output. The following example using the "reverse X" method will explain.

Example

Doctor order: 28% oxygen cold steam aerosol for high humidity.

Problem: The 28% setting produces a low density aerosol.

Solution: Place the nebulizer at the 40% setting and run the nebulizer off of a blender. The 40% setting will deliver a higher density aerosol and will still maintain a high flow rate of gas to the patient. If the blender is set at 100% the nebulizer will deliver 40%, but if the blender is set at less than 100% something less than 40% will be delivered.

Question: Where do you set the blender to deliver 28% to the patient?

Answer: The "reverse X" method (Figure 13-2). Place the desired FIO_2 in the middle of the X. Place the entrained gas (room air) oxygen concentration (21%) in the left arm of the X. Subtract the difference and place the number in the right leg of the X (in this case, 7). Since we are using the 40% setting, use the ratio of 3:1 and place the appropriate number in the right arm of the X. In this case a 3:1 ratio results in a 21:7 ratio ($3 \times 7 = 21$ and $1 \times 7 = 7$) where 7 is the number of liters of oxygen and 21 is the number of liters of air. Place 21 in the right arm of the X. Now add the right arm and middle number (21 + 28). This will give you 49. If the blender is set at 49%, and the nebulizer is set at the 40% dilution setting, 28% oxygen will be delivered by the nebulizer. This math assumes that everything is working perfectly, so always analyze the delivered mixture and tweak the knob as needed. Remember to label the set up with the actual FIO_2. Total flow will be determined by the flowmeter setting and the entrainment (ratio) setting. This process was

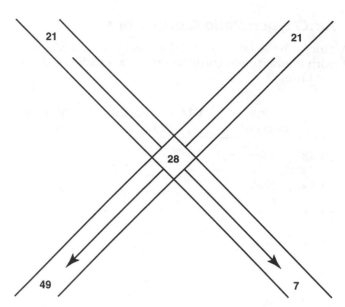

FIGURE 13-2. The reverse X method.

described earlier. If this whole process seems too confusing and too labor intensive, you may be correct. Maybe we should skip the aerosol and deliver a dry gas.

If you prefer, the V1C1 formula can also be used to determine the blender setting.

$$V1C1 + V2C2 = VtCt$$

Where:

V1 is the ratio value of room air (number depends on entrainment setting). In the above example, it is 3 since the 40% setting is used

C1 is the FIO_2 value of room air (always 21%)

V2 is the ratio value of the blender gas (always 1)

C2 is the FIO_2 of the blender gas (unknown)

Vt is the addition of the two ratio values (V1 + V2)

Ct is the desired FIO_2 you wish to deliver to the patient

Following the example above:

$$3 \times 0.21 + 1 \times ? = 4 \times 0.28$$
$$0.63 + ? = 1.12 \ ? = 0.49 \text{ or } 49\% \text{ for the blender setting}$$

Student Exercise

Using the methods described above, determine the required blender setting for each of the following cold steam setups.

	Desired FIO_2 (%)	Entrain-ment Setting (%)	Flow-meter Setting	Blender Setting	Total Flow
13-67.	24	40	12	_____	_____
13-68.	26	40	10	_____	_____
13-69.	28	50	12	_____	_____
13-70.	30	50	14	_____	_____
13-71.	40	35	8	_____	_____

REVIEW QUESTIONS

13-72. Each of the following are methods of oxygen production for patient use except:
A. fractional distillation of air
B. molecular sieve
C. electrolysis
D. membrane oxygen concentrator

13-73. Which of the following gases, when used with oxygen, may help a patient with increased airway resistance breathe easier?
A. helium
B. carbon dioxide
C. nitrogen
D. nitric oxide

13-74. Use of which of the following gases may help to decrease pulmonary vascular resistance?
A. helium
B. carbon dioxide
C. nitrogen
D. nitric oxide

13-75. Which of the following, when considered as a single entity, will result in hypoxemia but have a normal A-a gradient?
A. hypoventilation
B. $\dot{V}/\dot{Q}$ mismatch
C. shunting
D. diffusion defect

14

Hyperbaric Oxygen Therapy

Hyperbaric oxygen (HBO) therapy deals with the process of delivering gases under pressure. Associated clinical applications and hazards are listed in *Respiratory Care*. During the application of hyperbaric medicine, the relationships between pressure (P), volume (V), and temperature (T) are important considerations. A short review of these relationships is appropriate.

PRESSURE MEASUREMENTS

The pressure exerted by a gas is affected by the number of molecules present, the temperature of the system, and the volume of the container. Pressure can be measured by different methods; it can be expressed as atmospheric, gauge, or absolute pressure, and can be expressed in a variety of units. Atmospheric pressure (Patm) is the pressure exerted by the atmosphere and is measured with a barometer. Gauge pressure (Pga) is a pressure relative to Patm and is measured using a manometer. At one atmospheric pressure, gauge pressure is zero. Absolute pressure (Pabs), or total pressure, is the sum of gauge pressure and atmospheric pressure and is expressed in the following formula:

> Absolute pressure = atmospheric pressure + gauge pressure
>
> Pabs = Patm + Pga

Examples

> If Patm = 1034 cmH$_2$O, and Pga = 27 cmH$_2$O, Pabs = 1061 cmH$_2$O
>
> 1034 + 27 = 1061
> (pressure in an endotracheal tube cuff)

> If Pabs = 47 psi, and Patm = 14.7 psi, then Pga = 32.3 psi
>
> 47 − 14.7 = 32.3 (pressure in your car tires)

> If Pga = 120/80 mmHg, and Patm = 760 mmHg, then Pabs = 880/840 mmHg
> (pressure in your arterial blood vessels)

Pressure is force per unit surface area, yet force and nonforce units are often used to indicate pressure. Examples of force units include the following: psi (lb/in^2), dynes/cm^2, and g/cm^2. Examples of nonforce units include the following: mmHg, cmH$_2$O, and ftH$_2$O. It is commonly accepted to indicate pressure in the units of the height of a column of fluid since that column will result in a pressure. Many of the commonly used measurements to indicate 1 Patm are listed in Table 14-1.

Since each of the values listed in Table 14-1 is equal to 1 Patm, they are also equal to each other. Conversion from one unit to another can easily be made by using conversion factors. These factors can be derived by simply dividing one set of values into another.

TABLE 14-1 **Common Values and Units Used to Indicate 1 Patm at Sea Level**

760 mmHg
760 torr
76 cmHg
1034 cmH$_2$O
33.9 ft fresh water
33 fsw (ft of sea water)
14.7 psi
29.9 in Hg
101.3 kPa (kilopascal)
1.014×10^6 dynes/cm^2
1014 millibars
1034 g/cm^2

Examples

Factor to convert mmHg to cmH_2O

$$1034 \ cmH_2O/760 \ mmHg = 1.36 \ cmH_2O/mmHg$$

Factor to convert cm H_2O to ftH_2O (sea water)

$$33 \ ftH_2O/1034 \ cmH_2O = 0.032 \ ftH_2O/c \ H_2O$$

Factor to convert kPa to mmHg

$$760 \ mmHg/101.3 \ kPa = 7.5 \ mmHg/kPa$$

Pressure Conversions: Student Exercise

Develop the conversion factors for the following, then perform the following pressure conversions.

14-1. 700 mmHg to in Hg   _____

14-2. 800 mmHg to cmH_2O _____

14-3. 10 psi to mmHg   _____

14-4. 18 psi to cmH_2O _____

14-5. 80 fsw to no. of atms   _____

14-6. 20 kPa to mmHg   _____

14-7. 50 kPa to cmH_2O _____

14-8. 100 mmHg to kPa   _____

14-9. 100 cmH_2O to kPa   _____

14-10. 3.5 atms to fsw   _____

GAS LAWS

The temperature, pressure, and volume of a gas are interrelated. This relationship can be expressed in the following gas laws.

Boyle's Law

At a constant temperature (T), absolute pressure (P) exerted by a gas increases as the volume (V) decreases and vise versa. This relationship is expressed in the following formula:

$$P \times V = a \ constant$$

When starting with a given set of conditions (P1, V1) and then making a change in pressure or volume, yet keeping temperature constant, the formula to determine the new values (P2, V2) will be:

$$P1 \times V1 = P2 \times V2$$

Remember that pressure must be expressed as absolute pressure. If the final answer is to be expressed in gauge pressure, P2 will need to be converted appropriately.

During HBO, the application of Boyle's law is especially important during decompression. A loculated volume of gas will expand, and gas bubbles will form in solution if decompression occurs too rapidly. If this phenomenon occurs in a patient's body, it can result in complications, such as a pneumothorax, pulmonary gas emboli, tympanic membrane rupture, and sinus trauma.

Charles' Law

At a constant pressure (P), as volume (V) increases, absolute temperature (T) increases and visa versa. This relationship can be expressed in the following formula:

$$V/T = a \ constant$$

When starting with a given set of conditions (V1, T1) and then making a change in volume or temperature, yet keeping pressure constant, the formula to determine the new values (V2, T2) will be:

$$V1/T1 = V2/T2$$

Remember that temperature must be expressed in the absolute temperature scale of Kelvin. If the final answer is to be expressed in Celsius or Fahrenheit, T2 must be converted back to the appropriate temperature scale.

Gay-Lussac's Law

At a constant volume (V), as absolute temperature (T) increases, absolute pressure (P) increases and vise versa. This relationship can be expressed in the following formula:

$$P/T = a \text{ constant}$$

When starting with a given set of conditions (P1, T1) and then making a change in pressure or temperature, yet keeping volume constant, the formula to determine the new values (P2, T2) will be:

$$P1/T1 = P2/T2$$

Remember that both pressure and temperature must be expressed as absolute values in the formula.

Because the volume of the hyperbaric chamber is fixed, as P increases the T will also increase. This is an application of Gay-Lussac's law. For this reason, it is important to flush the chamber with air during pressurization to maintain an appropriate temperature.

Henry's Law

Henry's law is very important in a discussion dealing with HBO since many of the benefits associated with HBO are caused by the increased amount of O_2 that can be dissolved in the blood. The amount of oxygen that can dissolve in the blood is directly proportional to the partial pressure of oxygen in the alveoli and its solubility coefficient. The solubility of oxygen is 0.003 mL/dL of blood/mmHg pressure of oxygen. If the oxygen partial pressure is 1, then the amount of dissolved oxygen is as follows:

$$0.003 \times 1 = 0.003 \text{ mL/dL}$$

If the PO_2 is 100, then the dissolved oxygen is:

$$0.003 \times 100 = 0.3 \text{ mL/dL}$$

This is a normal PaO_2 and would result in a hemoglobin (Hb) saturation of 98%. If a person were to breathe 100% oxygen, and his or her lungs were normal, his or her PaO_2 may get as high as 600 to 620 mmHg. Although the PaO_2 value increases sixfold over a normal PaO_2, oxygen content does not. Since Hb is already 98% saturated at a PaO_2 of 100 mHg, lit-

tle oxygen can be added to the Hb. The only extra oxygen that enters the blood is in the dissolved state. Since the solubility coefficient is so low for oxygen, even increasing the PaO_2 to 600 does not add a large amount of oxygen to the total content.

Normal CaO_2 on room air: $0.003 \times 100 + 15 \times 0.98 \times 1.34 = 20.0$ mL/dL

CaO_2 breathing 100% O_2: $0.003 \times 600 + 15 \times 1.0 \times 1.34 = 21.9$ mL/dL

HBO therapy allows the PaO_2 to go to much higher levels. Let's quickly review the alveolar air equation.

$$P_{AO_2} = EBP \times F_{IO_2} - PaCO_2 \times 1.25$$

While breathing room air the alveolar oxygen is approximately 100 mmHg.

$$P_{AO_2} = 713 \times 0.21 - 40 \times 1.25 = \\ 150 - 50 = 100 \text{ mmHg}$$

While breathing 100% oxygen the alveolar oxygen is higher.

$$P_{AO_2} = 713 \times 1.0 - 40 = 713 - 40 = 673 \text{ mmHg}$$

When a patient is placed into a hyperbaric chamber, the equation must be modified to reflect the extra pressure. The following examples illustrate this point.

Examples

Example 1

Patient at 2 Patm on room air:

$$P_{AO_2} = (2 \times 760 - 47) \times 0.21 - 40 \times 1.25 = \\ 1473 \times 0.21 - 50 = 259 \text{ mmHg}$$

This is equivalent to breathing 43% oxygen. Where:

O_2 equivalent = $[P_{AO_2} + PaCO_2 \times 1.25]/EBP$ at 1 Patm

O_2 equivalent = $[259 + 40 \times 1.25]/713 = 309/713 = 0.43$

Example 2
Patient at 2 Patm on 100% oxygen:

$$P_{AO_2} = (2 \times 760 - 47) \times 1.0 - 40 = $$
$$1473 - 40 = 1433 \text{ mmHg}$$

This is an O_2 equivalent of 212% oxygen, which obviously cannot be obtained.

Example 3
Patient at 3 Patm on 100% oxygen:

$$P_{AO_2} = (3 \times 760 - 47) \times 1.0 - 40 = $$
$$2233 - 40 = 2193 \text{ mmHg}$$

Of course there are hazards associated with using high oxygen and pressure levels. These hazards are discussed in *Respiratory Care*. However, using high levels of oxygen and pressure does allow much more oxygen to be carried in the blood. If the P_{AO_2} is 2193 mmHg, the P_{aO_2} can be over 2000 mmHg. Now calculate CaO_2.

$$CaO_2 = (0.003 \times 2000) + (15 \times 1.0 \times 1.34)$$
$$CaO_2 = 6 + 20.1 = 26.1 \text{ mL } O_2/\text{dL blood}$$

One of the main purposes for using hyperbaric medicine for treatment of various conditions is to increase the O_2 dissolved in the plasma for ultimate delivery to cells. At this level of P_{aO_2}, it is possible for the plasma to supply all the O_2 needed for cellular function. Oxygen on the hemoglobin need not be unloaded. In theory, and in actual practice, a person would not need Hb for O_2 delivery at this level of P_{aO_2}.

One final note. As of this writing, the use of HBO therapy is becoming very popular for treatment of soft-tissue sport injuries. Whether or not it will prove to be a justified reason for HBO use is yet to be seen.

DIVING AND HYPERBARICS

Divers are affected by the same principles of hyperbarics. Since divers do not require high P_{aO_2} levels, they can avoid some of the risks involved with hyperbaric medicine by breathing He/O_2 mixtures (with less than 21% O_2) for deep dives and for long submersion periods. Breathing He/O_2 mixtures decreases the chances of both pulmonary and systemic O_2 toxicity. The decreased density of an He/O_2 mixture also makes breathing easier (decreases resistance to flow) compared with breathing room air. This is an application of Poiseuille's law for turbulent flow.

HYPOBARIC CONDITIONS

Although the objective of this chapter is to discuss HBO, it is important to mention hypobaric conditions (pressures less than one normal atmospheric pressure). Routinely, pressures less than 1 Patm are acutely experienced when ascending to high altitudes during flight, or driving up a mountain such as Pikes Peak in Colorado. It is chronically experienced by those who live at high altitudes. Ascent to high altitudes results in decompression, and the principles and hazards described with decompression from hyperbaric conditions apply. However, the magnitude is usually less. Both acute ascents and high-altitude dwelling result in P_{AO_2} and P_{aO_2} values lower than the "normal" values owing to the atmospheric pressure being less than the 760 mmHg at sea level. If blood oxygen levels drop significantly, hypoxemia can result. This can cause hyperventilation and acute altitude sickness, which is often manifested by headache, fatigue, dizziness, nausea, loss of appetite, and palpitations.

Student Exercises

Calculate the P_{AO_2} and the O_2 equivalent for each of the following:

	Patm	FIO_2	P_{AO_2} (mmHg)	O_2 Equiv (%)
14-11.	0.5	.50	_____	_____
14-12.	0.75	.50	_____	_____
14-13.	1.5	.50	_____	_____
14-14.	1.5	1.0	_____	_____
14-15.	2.0	.50	_____	_____
14-16.	2.5	.50	_____	_____
14-17.	3.0	.21	_____	_____

Calculate the total CaO_2 for the following:

	PaO_2 (mmHg)	Hb (g)	O_2Sat (%)	CaO_2 (mL/dL)
14-18.	30	15	55	_____
14-19.	80	8	96	_____
14-20.	1200	8	100	_____
14-21.	60	12	90	_____
14-22.	2000	12	100	_____
14-23.	100	5	100	_____
14-24.	2000	5	100	_____
14-25.	2200	0	0	_____

REVIEW QUESTIONS

14-26. A patient in an HBO chamber is breathing compressed air at an absolute pressure of 1600 mmHg. What is the oxygen equivalent?
A. 32%
B. 39%
C. 46%
D. 52%

14-27. Hazards associated with HBO therapy include all of the following except:
A. fire
B. barotrauma
C. low humidity
D. high noise levels

14-28. Which of the following is an absolute contraindication to HBO therapy?
A. pregnancy
B. emphysema
C. untreated pneumothorax
D. optic neuritis

14-29. Which of the following is equal to 2 Patm?
A. 14.7 psig
B. 760 mmHg (barometric pressure)
C. 1034 cmH$_2$O (Pabs)
D. 66 fsw (gauge)

14-30. Complications of HBO therapy include all of the following except:
A. increased work of breathing
B. atelectasis
C. cerebral oxygen toxicity
D. cooling during the pressurization phase (the dive)

14-31. Mechanical ventilators used in an HBO chamber should be:
A. pressure cycled
B. volume cycled
C. time cycled
D. flow cycled

14-32. Approved indications for HBO therapy include all of the following except:
A. carbon monoxide poisoning
B. radiation tissue damage
C. gas gangrene
D. sports injuries

14-33. A mountain climber is at an elevation where the PIO_2 is 80 mmHg and his PAO_2 is 50 mmHg. What is his oxygen equivalent?
A. 8%
B. 11%
C. 14%
D. 17%

15

Humidity and Aerosol Therapy

HUMIDITY

Water Vapor Pressure and Water Vapor Content

Just as other gases in a gas mixture each exert a partial pressure, water vapor pressure (PH_2O) is the pressure exerted by molecular water (water vapor) that has evaporated into the atmosphere. If a gas is completely dry, there is no water vapor or water vapor pressure. The maximum amount of molecular water that can be present in a gas sample is directly related to the temperature of the gas. The water vapor pressure is directly related to the actual amount of molecular water present in a sample. It is important to note that PH_2O does not change as total system pressure changes, and from this standpoint does not follow Dalton's law as true gases do. It is also the reason why PH_2O is always subtracted from the barometric pressure in the alveolar air equation before multiplying by the FIO_2. Table 15-1 lists various temperatures, the maximum mg/L of water present, and the PH_2O at that level of content.

Each of the values listed in Table 15-1 are at the maximum water content in molecular form (water vapor content, WVC) for the given temperature (the gas is completely saturated). This is also known as 100% relative humidity (RH). RH is the ratio of the actual (absolute, content) amount of molecular water present divided by the potential (capacity, maximum) amount of molecular water that could be present.

TABLE 15-1 **Water Vapor Content and PH_2O at 100% RH for a Given Temperature**

Temperature (°C)	Water Vapor Content (mg/L)	PH_2O (mmHg)
0	4.8	4.6
5	6.8	6.5
10	9.4	9.2
15	12.8	12.8
16	13.6	13.6
17	14.5	14.5
18	15.4	15.5
19	16.3	16.5
20	17.3	17.5
21	18.4	18.7
22	19.4	19.8
23	20.6	21.1
24	21.8	22.4
25	23.0	23.8
26	24.4	25.2
27	25.8	26.7
28	27.2	28.4
29	28.8	30.0
30	30.4	31.8
31	32.0	33.7
32	33.8	35.7
33	35.6	37.7
34	37.6	39.9
35	39.6	42.2
36	41.7	44.6
37	43.9	47.1
38	46.2	49.7
39	48.6	52.4
40	51.1	55.3
100	598.0	760.0

Example 1
At 37°C the potential humidity is 43.9 mg/L. If the actual humidity is also 43.9 mg/L, the RH is 100%. RH = (43.9/43.9) × 100 = 100%. The PH_2O is 47 mmHg based on the actual 43.9 mg/L present.

Example 2
If at 37°C only 21.95 mg/L of water is present, the RH is 50% since the potential is still 43.9 mg/L. RH = (21.95/43.9) × 100 = 50%. The PH_2O, in this case, is only approximately 23 mmHg since the PH_2O is based on the actual water vapor present.

Example 3
If at 24°C the gas has a RH of 50%, the amount of water present is 11.9 mg/L (0.5 × 21.8 = 11.9).

Calculation of Water Vapor Content and PH₂O

Using Table 15-1, determine the WVC and PH₂O given the following information.

	Temperature (°C)	%RH	WVC (mg/t)	PH₂O (mmHg)
15-1.	16	100	____	____
15-2.	16	50	____	____
15-3.	20	40	____	____
15-4.	20	80	____	____
15-5.	24	100	____	____
15-6.	24	25	____	____
15-7.	37	35	____	____
15-8.	37	75	____	____

Calculation of Relative Humidity

Using Table 15-1, determine the potential humidity and RH given the following information.

	Temperature (°C)	Actual Humidity (mg/L)	Potential Humidity (mg/L)	%RH
15-9.	18	11	____	____
15-10.	22	6	____	____
15-11.	24	17	____	____
15-12.	24	5	____	____
15-13.	30	15	____	____
15-14.	37	27	____	____
15-15.	37	38	____	____

HUMIDIFIERS

The maximum amount of water vapor a gas can hold is directly related to the temperature of the gas. Unheated humidifiers, regardless of their style of construction, are very inefficient because they deliver gas at or below room temperature owing to the cooling effect of evaporation. Heated humidifiers are very efficient since they can be heated to or above body temperature when delivering humidity.

Laboratory Exercises

15-16. Select several humidifiers, both heated and unheated, and compare their construction and method of operation. Which of the humidifiers have pressure release valves? Test them to document the pop-off pressure level.

15-17. Select one unheated humidifier and fill it with water. Allow it to stand for a period of time so it can equilibrate with room temperature. Document the temperature. Bubble oxygen through the humidifier at various flow rates, documenting the change in temperatures as flow rate is changed. How will this change in temperature affect the humidity output of the humidifier?

15-18. Select one humidifier and place a known volume of water into the humidifier. Bubble oxygen through it at a known flow rate for a known period of time. After several hours, determine the amount of water that evaporated by subtracting the remaining volume from the initial volume. Determine the milligrams of water per liter of gas by dividing the total water output by the total number of liters of gas that passed through the humidifier. Also determine %RH by dividing this actual water output by the potential humidity at the measured temperature. This exercise can be carried out for both heated and unheated humidifiers.

NEBULIZERS

Nebulizers differ from humidifiers in that they deliver a gas to patients containing both molecular water and water particles (an aerosol). Nebulizers vary in their efficiency in delivering aerosols. Some nebulizers have a very poor aerosol output and do not provide enough humidity to deliver 100% RH at body temperature. Others can deliver well over 100% RH at body conditions (43.9 mg/L).

Example

Using a commercially available pneumatic jet nebulizer, we did an experiment to test for water output at several oxygen dilution settings. On the 28% dilution setting, we delivered 450 mL of water in 235 minutes. The output from the nebulizer was 1.91 mL/min (450/235). Since we used the 28% dilution setting, the ratio of air to oxygen was 10:1. The flowmeter setting was 14 L/min. The total flow through the device was 154 L/min (14 × 11) and 36,190 L total (154 ×

235). The density of the output can be calculated by dividing the milliliters of water output by the total number of liters of flow: 450 mL/36,190 L = 0.01243 mL water/L of gas. Since 1 mL = 1 g = 1000 mg, density was 12.43 mg/L.

At the 40% dilution setting, we delivered 450 mL in 455 minutes. Output was 0.99 mL/min, (450/455). Total flow was 56 L/min (4 × 14) and 25,480 L (56 × 455). Density was 450/25,480 or 17.66 mg/L.

At the 60% dilution setting, we delivered 450 mL in 535 minutes. Output was 0.84 mL/min (450/535). Total flow was 28 L/min (2 × 14) and 14,980 L (28 × 535). Density was 450/14,980 or 30.04 mg/L.

These values indicate that water output per minute is greater at low dilution settings, but because total flow is so much higher at low dilution settings, the density of that output is lower at low dilution settings. Remember that 43.9 mg/L is needed to completely humidify inspired gas to body conditions. The nebulizer that was tested fell well below this value at all dilution settings. Finally, the density, as listed, includes both molecular and particulate water output from the nebulizer's water reservoir, but it does not include the molecular water that was present in the environment. Since the nebulizer entrained room air, it also entrained the humidity present in room air. This humidity would have also been delivered to the patient, but it does not show up on the calculations. If this factor was to be considered, the density values of the mgH_2O/L of gas would most likely be higher than reported here.

Laboratory Exercises

15-19. Obtain several types of nebulizers: pneumatic and electrical, jet, and Babington styles. Compare their construction and methods of operation.

15-20. Select a nebulizer and fill it with a known volume of water. Power the nebulizer with a predetermined flow and entrainment setting. (Analyze it to make sure it is accurate.) After several hours, determine the amount of water nebulized by subtracting the amount left in the nebulizer from the initial volume. Calculate the total flow for the given time period the nebulizer was operating. Divide the milligrams of water nebulized by the total flow in liters. The result will be the density (mg/L) of the aerosol. Repeat this exercise for several different types of aerosol generators and compare their outputs. Which are able to deliver at least 43.9 mg/L?

%RH at Body Temperature

Although %RH can be calculated at any temperature, the actual amount of water present is often compared with what is needed to completely humidify a gas at body temperature. If the water content is 11.9 mg/L of gas at 24°C, the RH is 50% (11.9/21.8). If we want

to know what the RH would be at body temperature, we divide the 11.9 by 43.9 since that is what is needed at 37°C (11.9/43.9 = 27% RH).

Calculation of RH at Body Temperature

Using the values from 15-9 to 15-13, determine the %RH at body temperature based on the actual humidity (AH) present. Compare these values with the %RH calculated in 15-9 to 15-13 for the given temperature.

15-21. AH from 15-9. = 11 mg/L _____ %RH at 37°C

15-22. AH from 15-10. = 6 mg/L _____ %RH at 37°C

15-23. AH from 15-11. = 17 mg/L _____ %RH at 37°C

15-24. AH from 15-12. = 5 mg/L _____ %RH at 37°C

15-25. AH from 15-13. = 15 mg/L _____ %RH at 37°C

HUMIDITY DEFICIT

Humidity deficit (HD) is the difference between the actual amount of water delivered per liter of gas compared with the amount that is needed at 37°C and 100% RH. If the amount of water delivered is less than 43.9 mg/L, the deficit must be made up by evaporation of water from the subject's airways. This is a normal phenomena for all of us, but in intubated patients, a large humidity deficit may lead to drying of secretions and other pulmonary complications. HD is calculated by subtracting the actual amount of water present in a gas sample from 43.9 mg/L.

Example

A nasal cannula is being used to deliver oxygen at 2 L/min. The oxygen is flowing through a bubble humidifier. The temperature of the gas exiting the humidifier is 20°C and is measured to be 80% RH. The actual amount of water present is 80% of 17.3 mg/L (0.8 × 17.3 = 13.84 mg/L). HD is equal to 43.9 − 13.84 or 30.06 mg/L.

With low-flow systems and entrainment devices, the source gas accounts for only part of the total inspired gas volume, and room air makes up the rest. It is probably not as important to correct humidity deficit for these devices as it is for devices that deliver the total volume to the subject. It is also not as critical to correct a humidity deficit for a patient who still has his or her normal upper airway intact compared with one that is bypassed with an endotracheal tube.

Calculation of Humidity Deficit

Given the following information, calculate the HD.

15-26. 18°C   33% RH   _____ mg/L HD

15-27. 20°C   60% RH   _____ mg/L HD

15-28. 25°C   0% RH   _____ mg/L HD

15-29. 30°C   40% RH   _____ mg/L HD

15-30. 35°C   80% RH   _____ mg/L HD

REVIEW QUESTIONS

15-31. Inspired gas is normally at BTPS conditions by the time it reaches:
A. the nasopharynx
B. the vocal cords
C. the carina
D. the segmental bronchi

15-32. The water vapor pressure at 37°C and 100% RH is:
A. 24 mmHg
B. 37 mmHg
C. 44 mmHg
D. 47 mmHg

15-33. A device used to warm and humidify inspired gases by collecting exhaled heat and moisture is the:
A. bubbler
B. wick
C. heat and moisture exchanger (HME)
D. cascade

15-34. Which of the following is the most important reason as to why low-flow bubble humidifiers are limited in their ability to deliver humidity?
A. their short height
B. their lack of ability to create small bubbles
C. the fact that they are unheated
D. short contact time

15-35. Approximately what percent of particles from clinical nebulizers are retained in the lungs of nonintubated subjects?
A. 2%–3%
B. 10%–12%
C. 19%–21%
D. 42%–46%

15-36. The amount of water present in normal alveolar gas is:
A. 38 mg/L
B. 40 mg/L
C. 44 mg/L
D. 47 mg/L

15-37. Compared with unheated humidifiers, a major advantage of heated humidifiers is that:
A. particles are produced in the therapeutic range
B. both molecular and particulate water are produced
C. a baffle is not needed
D. 100% RH is easily attained at body temperature

15-38. The humidity deficit of a patient, with a normal body temperature, breathing gas that is at 57% RH at 37°C is:
A. 16.2 mg/L
B. 18.8 mg/L
C. 20.2 mg/L
D. 24.7 mg/L

16

Drugs Used in Respiratory Care

Drugs are used for many reasons. Some help to regulate organs and organ systems. Some help to reduce pain. Some fight infections, and others help prevent clotting of blood. Drugs are also important for helping to relax bronchial smooth muscle and decrease airway inflammation. This latter category is the subject of this chapter.

DRUG ADMINISTRATION

Drugs can be administered by several routes. Enteral administration (by mouth) is very common. Parenteral administration normally includes injections, such as subcutaneous, intramuscular, and intravenous. Topical and transcutaneous routes are also used. Finally, the inhaled route can be used and is the common pathway for administration of respiratory care medications.

TERMINOLOGY

A few terms are discussed as they relate to respiratory care drugs.

Potency: Potency compares the effect of one drug with another based on the amount of drug used to achieve a desired effect. If drug A (using 1 g) compared with drug B (using 10 g) achieves the same effect, drug A is more potent.

Intrinsic activity: Intrinsic activity is a comparison of drugs to see which can cause the greatest effect regardless of dosage. Varied potency and intrinsic effects help explain why varied doses of drugs are used.

Tachyphylaxis and tolerance: Over a period of time, the same dose of a drug may result in less effect. This results in the need to increase the drug dose or to change to another drug. If this phenomenon happens over a long period of time, it is called tolerance. If it happens quickly, it is called tachyphylaxis.

Additive: When two drugs, given together, have an effect equal to the sum of the individual effects, their relationship is said to be additive (1 + 1 = 2).

Synergistic: When two drugs, given together, have an effect greater than the sum of their individual effects, their relationship is said to be synergistic (1 + 1 = 3).

Potentiation: When two drugs, given together, have an effect greater than the sum of their individual effects, and one of the drugs normally by itself has no effect, their relationship is said to be one of potentiation (1 + 0 = 2).

DRUG SOLUTIONS

Common respiratory drug solutions are based on a weight/volume relationship, where weight is in grams (g) and volume is in milliliters (mL). A mixture of 2 g of drug in 100 mL of solution is a 2% solution. A mixture with 10 g of drug in 100 mL of solution is a 10% solution. A 0.3% solution has 0.3 g of drug in 100 mL of solution. A mixture with 5 g of drug in 20 mL of solution is a 25% solution. This last one would have the same concentration as 25 g in 100 mL of solution.

Problem Set

Calculate the percent solutions for each of the following.

	Grams of Drug	Milliliters of Solution	Percent Solution
16-1.	1	100	_____
16-2.	3	300	_____
16-3.	1	10	_____
16-4.	5	100	_____
16-5.	2	50	_____
16-6.	10	50	_____
16-7.	0.5	100	_____

Examples of the Relationship Between Milligrams, Milliliters, and Percent Solution

Example 1

Given the percent solution and the number of milliliters of solution, the number of milligrams of drug present can be calculated.

0.5 mL of a 2% solution will contain how many mg of drug?

$$2\% = \frac{2\,g}{100\,mL} = \frac{2000\,mg}{100\,mL} = \frac{X\,mg}{0.5\,mL} \quad X = 10\,mg$$

Example 2

Given the percent solution and the number of milligrams of drug desired, the required amount of solution (mL) can be calculated.

How many milliliters of a 5% solution are needed to give 40 mg of a drug?

$$5\% = \frac{5\,g}{100\,mL} = \frac{5000\,mg}{100\,mL} = \frac{40\,mg}{X\,mL} \quad X = 0.8\,mL$$

Example 3

Given the milligrams of drug present and the milliliters of drug present, the percent solution can be calculated.

What is the percent solution if 30 mg of drug is present in 0.5 mL of solution?

$$\frac{30\,mg}{0.5\,mL} = \frac{60\,mg}{1\,mL} = \frac{6000\,mg}{100\,mL} = \frac{6\,g}{100\,mL} = 6\%\ solution$$

Example 4

If 1 mL of a 3% solution is mixed with 3 mL of saline, how many mg of drug are present, and what is the final percent solution after mixing?

$$3\% = \frac{3\,g}{100\,mL} = \frac{3000\,mg}{100\,mL} = \frac{30\,mg}{1\,mL}$$

You are starting out with 30 mg. This same amount of drug remains after mixing but you now have 4 mL of solution.

$$\frac{30\,mg}{4\,mL} = \frac{750\,mg}{100\,mL} = \frac{0.75\,g}{100\,mL} = 0.75\%\ solution$$

Calculation Exercises

16-8.   Given 0.25 mL of a 1% solution, calculate the milligrams of drug present.

16-9.   Given a 2% solution, calculate the number of milliliters of solution that will contain 40 mg of drug.

16-10. 0.5 mL of solution containing 50 mg of drug is mixed with 2 mL of H_2O, what is the final percent solution?

16-11. How would you prepare 50 mL of a 5% NaCl solution?

16-12. How many grams of Alupent are there in a 20-mL bottle of 5% solution?

16-13. How many grams of dextrose are in 250 mL of a 5% dextrose solution?

16-14. A patient is to be given 0.3 mL of a 5% Alupent solution by aerosol. How many milligrams of drug will be delivered?

16-15. A patient is to be given 0.5 mL of a 0.5% albuterol solution by aerosol. How many milligrams of drug will be delivered?

16-16. Show that 0.5 mL of a 0.5% solution of albuterol (multidose vial) has the same number of milligrams of drug as 3 mL of a 0.083% solution of albuterol (unit dose).

REVIEW QUESTIONS

16-17. Advantages of aerosol therapy include all of the following except:
    A. relatively small amounts of drug can be given
    B. onset of action is slow
    C. minimal systemic side effects
    D. relatively frequent doses can be given with little chance of toxicity

16-18. The typical patient given an aerosol will deposit approximately what percent of the drug in the respiratory tract?
    A. 1%–2%
    B. 5%–10%
    C. 20%–25%
    D. 45%–55%

16-19. Infected sputum would most likely appear:
    A. brown
    B. red
    C. green or yellow
    D. white

16-20. All of the following are correct concerning acetylcysteine (Mucomyst) except:
    A. it is a respiratory tract irritant and may induce bronchospasm
    B. it will stimulate ciliary activity
    C. it may cause nausea
    D. it ruptures the disulfide bridges of mucoprotein

16-21. Which of the following drugs may help a newborn decrease its chance of developing respiratory distress syndrome of the newborn?
A. pulmozyme
B. ribavirin
C. sodium bicarb
D. exosurf

16-22. The most frequent and important reason for administering aerosol agents is to:
A. relieve bronchospasm
B. cause vasoconstriction
C. cause local anesthesia
D. fight infection

16-23. Albuterol is classified as a:
A. steroid
B. parasympatholytic
C. mucolytic
D. sympathomimetic

16-24. Which of the following is not classified as a bronchodilator?
A. Atrovent
B. Alupent
C. Intal
D. Isuprel

16-25. Albuterol causes relaxation of smooth muscle by increasing the intracellular level of which of the following?
A. cyclic 3,5-AMP
B. phosphodiesterase
C. cyclic 3,5-GMP
D. carbonic anhydrase

16-26. Epinephrine can be classified as each of the following except:
A. sympathomimetic
B. beta agonist
C. adrenoreceptor stimulant
D. cholinergic agent

16-27. Stimulation of beta-2 sites throughout the body will result in each of the following except:
A. bronchodilation
B. vasodilation
C. tachycardia
D. tremor

16-28. All of the following decrease theophylline clearance rate except:
A. hypoxia
B. smoking
C. venous congestion
D. hepatocellular failure

16-29. If a seemingly large dose of drug is ordered for aerosol administration, the therapist should:
A. flatly refuse to deliver it
B. discuss it with the doctor
C. deliver the medication without question
D. give a treatment, but substitute the normal dose of drug

17

Bronchial Hygiene Therapy

Bronchial hygiene therapy (BHT) involves the use of various techniques or devices to aid in the removal of airway secretions. Unlike many of the therapies with which respiratory care practitioners are involved, BHT can often be conducted without mechanical aids. That means these techniques can be used just about anywhere and at any time without expensive equipment.

Student Exercises

17-1. List six precautions/contraindications for postural drainage therapy techniques.

a. _____

b. _____

c. _____

d. _____

e. _____

f. _____

17-2. List the four treatment objectives of breathing exercises.

a. _____

b. _____

c. _____

d. _____

Laboratory Exercises

For each of the following, select a partner and practice the breathing exercises. This exercise will allow opportunity for instruction as well as actually experiencing the various maneuvers. Take turns explaining and doing the exercises.

17-3. Controlled deep breathing: As per your instruction, have your partner alter their breathing rate, pattern, and volume.

17-4. Active cycle of breathing (ACB): Following the guidelines in box 17-8 of *Respiratory Care*, encourage each other to perform the ACB exercises as outlined. Note that the forced expiratory technique is not a cough but a "huff." That is, a forced exhalation but not against a closed glottis.

17-5. Autogenic drainage: Practice autogenic drainage as outlined in Figure 17-3 of *Respiratory Care*.

17-6. Postural drainage therapy: Practice postural drainage therapy by positioning your partner to maximize drainage for the different pulmonary segments.

17-7. Percussion and vibration: Practice percussion and vibration, using both manual (your hands) and mechanical techniques if mechanical percussors are available.

17-8. Directed cough: Practice direct cough "gently" on each other as outlined in *Respiratory Care*.

REVIEW QUESTIONS

17-9. The primary goal of BHT is which of the following?
A. increase exercise tolerance
B. remove excessive airway secretions
C. decrease supplemental oxygen use
D. decrease hospital stay

17-10. The single most important factor preventing the retention of secretions is:
A. the cough
B. pursed lip breathing
C. ciliary motion
D. chest physical therapy

17-11. Ventilatory muscle fatigue will be indicated by all of the following except:
A. diaphragmatic breathing
B. tachypnea
C. use of accessory muscles
D. thoraco-abdominal dyssynchrony

17-12. The silhouette sign refers to which of the following?
A. the heart shadow on a radiograph
B. the hilar markings on a radiograph
C. the position of the diaphragm on a radiograph
D. the obliteration of normal contrast on a radiograph

17-13. To maximize oxygenation, the patient with unilateral lung disease should be positioned:
A. prone
B. supine
C. good lung down
D. bad lung down

18

Volume Expansion Therapy

Volume expansion therapy includes several types of procedures important for aiding in preventing atelectasis and removing secretions. The therapies discussed in *Respiratory Care* include incentive spirometry, intermittent positive pressure breathing (IPPB), continuous positive airway pressure (CPAP), positive expiratory pressure (PEP), expiratory positive airway pressure (EPAP), blow bottles, high-frequency airway oscillation, and high-frequency chest wall compression. These therapies and the devices used to deliver them provide a foundation for many of the procedures a respiratory care practitioner (RCP) will perform.

Obtain several types of incentive spirometry devices.

Evaluate each device as to its mode of operation: volume displacement or flow oriented.

Which of the devices record the number of attempts or record the attempts that reach the desired goal?

What type of incentive is used to help the patient maintain an sustained maximal inspiration (SMI)?

Breathe through each device. Give a subjective rating as to ease of breathing. Does one device increase the work of breathing over another?

Role play, teaching a fellow student to perform an incentive spirometry treatment. What will happen if your patient breathes through his or her nose or has a leak around his or her lips? How can this be corrected?

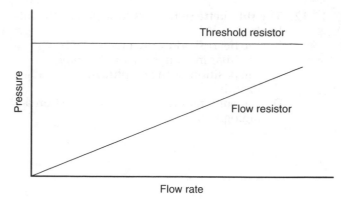

FIGURE 18-1. *Graph illustrating the change in pressure as flow rate changes for both threshold resistors and flow resistors.*

RESISTORS

There are two basic types of resistors, the threshold resistor and the flow resistor. The threshold resistor, or variable orifice resistor as some wish to call it, will automatically allow excess flow to pass through it without creating a higher system pressure. An ideal threshold resistor will maintain a constant system pressure regardless of the amount of flow through the system. A threshold resistor will maintain pressure in the system even when flow has stopped.

The flow resistor, or fixed orifice resistor, will not allow excess flow to pass through it without an increase in system pressure. Some flow resistors may have a manual adjustment to allow extra flow to exit the valve, thus allowing different pressure settings at different flow rates. Flow and pressure are directly proportional with a flow resistor. As flow increases, pressure increases. As flow deceases, pressure decreases. With a pure flow resistor, system pressure will drop to zero if flow stops. Figure 18-1 demonstrates the relationship between pressure and flow for each type of resistor. Some (many) valves end up acting as a hybrid, not totally following the ideal threshold or flow resistor pattern.

Resistors

Obtain several types of resistors. Set up a system allowing an inlet for flow and an outlet for flow through the resistor. Place a manometer proximal to the resistor. Also place a test lung in line so that the resistor can create end-expiratory pressure (EEP) for the lung. For each resistor to be tested, set the system pressure at 10 cmH$_2$O by initially adjusting the resistor or the flow as needed. Once set, increase the flow in increments of 10 L/min. Measure the system pressure for each change in flow. Does the resistor behave more like a threshold resistor or a flow resistor?

Flow (Initial L/min)	Resistor 1 (10 cmH$_2$O)	Resistor 2 (10 cmH$_2$O)	Resistor 3 (10 cmH$_2$O)
↑ 10	___ cmH$_2$O	___ cmH$_2$O	___ cmH$_2$O
↑ 20	___ cmH$_2$O	___ cmH$_2$O	___ cmH$_2$O
↑ 30	___ cmH$_2$O	___ cmH$_2$O	___ cmH$_2$O
↑ 40	___ cmH$_2$O	___ cmH$_2$O	___ cmH$_2$O
↑ 50	___ cmH$_2$O	___ cmH$_2$O	___ cmH$_2$O
↑ 60	___ cmH$_2$O	___ cmH$_2$O	___ cmH$_2$O
↑ 70	___ cmH$_2$O	___ cmH$_2$O	___ cmH$_2$O

CPAP

Set up a CPAP system. Have a variety of CPAP valves available for use. At a low CPAP level, breathe through the system, then exchange one CPAP valve for another. Note the subjective work of breathing and the fluctuations in pressure as a result of using different valves, at different flow rates and at different pressures.

PURSED LIP BREATHING

Normally, inspiration is an active maneuver. It requires muscle contraction, consumes oxygen, and uses energy. Normal exhalation is passive. It occurs as the chest muscles relax and the lungs recoil to their resting position at functional residual capacity (FRC). Figures 18-2 through 18-5 illustrate the lung and thoracic pressures during the normal inspiratory and expiratory cycles. The numbers used are for discussion purposes only, actual values will vary. Zero pressure is atmospheric, a "+" indicates pressure higher than atmospheric pressure, and a "−" indicates pressure lower than atmospheric.

Individuals with chronic obstructive pulmonary disease (COPD) have floppy airways that tend to collapse during exhalation. Secretions, bronchospasm, and airway edema may also create airflow obstruction. Each of these factors increase airflow resistance during exhalation and may result in increased work of breathing (WOB), shortness of breath (SOB), and air trapping (alveolar air trapped in the lung). Both inspiration and expiration can become active maneuvers, and energy must be expended during both respiratory cycles. This active breathing also results in pressure changes within the thorax. During exhalation, pleural pressures become positive and squeeze the airway. In normal lungs, this happens only during forced exhalation. When pleural pressure equals the pressure in the airway, a point called the equal pressure point (EPP) is reached. At this point and at all points exposed to the positive pressure down-

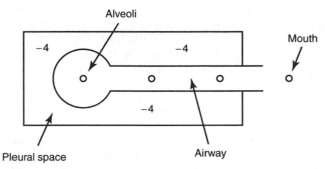

FIGURE 18-2. Resting level of breathing at FRC with no air movement and glottis open. With no air movement, pressures are equal along the airway.

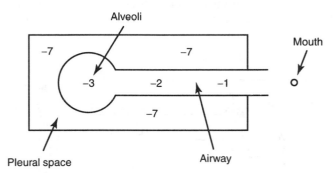

FIGURE 18-3. Active inspiration (normal breathing). Air flows as a result of a pressure gradient. For air to enter the lungs, pressure must be lower in the alveoli than it is at the mouth.

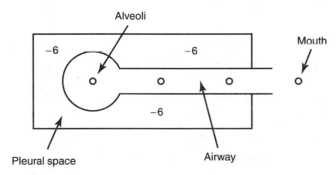

FIGURE 18-4. Inspiratory pause at end inspiration with glottis open. With no air movement, pressures along the airway are equal.

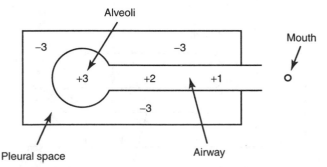

FIGURE 18-5. Passive exhalation (normal breathing). To allow air to exit the lungs, alveolar pressure must be greater than mouth pressure.

stream (closer to the mouth), the airway will be compressed. Larger airways being more rigid may have minimal compression, but small airways will collapse. Figures 18-6 and 18-7 illustrate the pressures during inspiration and exhalation in the thorax for an individual with COPD.

Pursed lip breathing may help relieve some of this compression. Pursing the lips (hold your lips in a position similar to when you whistle) creates back pressure in the airway during exhalation, thus helping to splint the airway open. Figure 18-8 illustrates the pursed lip effect.

Creating back pressure by pursing the lips helps to move the EPP downstream into a larger airway which is less likely to collapse. Thus, the patient is able to exhale a greater amount of air, reducing air trapping and allowing for better gas distribution breath after breath.

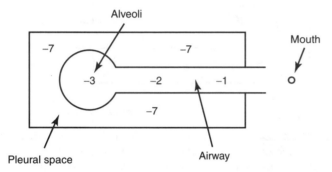

FIGURE 18-6. *Inspiration in patients with COPD.*

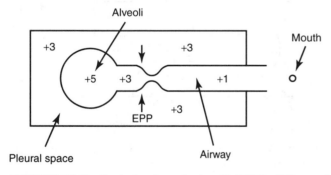

FIGURE 18-7. *Expiration in patients with COPD. EPP, equal pressure point.*

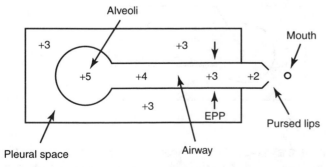

FIGURE 18-8. *Pressure changes with pursed lip breathing.*

REVIEW QUESTIONS

18-1. Each of the following are signs of atelectasis except:
   A. increased radiographic density
   B. elevation of contralateral diaphragm
   C. mediastinal shift toward affected side
   D. hyperinflation of surrounding segments

18-2. Atelectasis is associated with each of the following except:
   A. pulmonary shunt
   B. hypoxemia
   C. fever
   D. decreased compliance

18-3. Risk factors for developing atelectasis include each of the following except:
   A. retained secretions
   B. pain following upper abdominal surgery
   C. prolonged supine position
   D. frequent repositioning of patient

18-4. A patient should be turned or repositioned a minimum of every how many hours?
   A. 1 hour
   B. 2 hours
   C. 3 hours
   D. 4 hours

18-5. Complications of IPPB would include all of the following except:
   A. barotrauma
   B. increased cardiac output
   C. nosocomial infection
   D. gastric distention

18-6. A positive pressure will most likely be maintained during both inspiration and expiration in which of the following?
   A. CPAP
   B. EPAP
   C. PEP
   D. IPPB

18-7. Which of the following resistors would have the greatest pressure change as flow changes?
   A. magnetic valve
   B. weighted ball
   C. fixed orifice device
   D. spring-loaded valve

18-8. PEEP and CPAP have been shown to be effective in all of the following except:
   A. therapeutic use in nonintubated patients
   B. increasing the alveolar-arterial oxygen tension difference
   C. reducing intrapulmonary shunt
   D. increasing FRC

18-9. A patient experiencing light-headedness following an incentive spirometry treatment is most likely suffering from which of the following?
   A. pneumothorax
   B. hyperventilation

C. carbon dioxide retention

D. hypoxemia

18-10. Each of the following are goals of PAP therapy except:

A. to increase air trapping

B. aid in mobilization of secretions

C. prevent or reverse atelectasis

D. optimize delivery of bronchodilators

18-11. Contraindications of PAP may include all of the following except:

A. hemodynamic instability

B. decreased intracranial pressure < 20 mmHg

C. recent hemoptysis

D. untreated pneumothorax

18-12. A threshold resistor is set to maintain 10 cmH_2O at a flow of 30 L/min. What will happen to the system pressure if flow is increased to 50 L/min?

A. increase

B. decrease

C. no change

18-13. A flow resistor is set to maintain 10 cmH_2O at a flow of 30 L/min. What will happen to the system pressure if flow is increased to 50 L/min?

A. increase

B. decrease

C. no change

19

Airway Management

Airway management is very important in both basic life support and advanced life support. Techniques and equipment used in airway management are discussed in Chapter 19 of *Respiratory Care*. The following exercises and questions review some of that material.

LABORATORY EXERCISES

19-1. Using a mannequin, demonstrate at least two techniques for establishment of an airway in an unconscious victim. Now practice mask, bag-valve-mask, and face shield ventilation.

19-2. Using a mannequin, demonstrate the proper technique for inserting and securing of each of the following: oropharyngeal airway, nasopharyngeal airway, oral endotube, nasal endotube, and esophageal airway.

19-3. Obtain several different laryngoscope handles and blades and perform the following:
1. Compare and classify their construction
2. Disassemble and correctly reassemble each
3. Demonstrate proper use of each for intubation

19-4. Obtain several endotracheal (ET) and tracheostomy tubes and identify all markings and structures present. How does a Magill ET tube differ from a Murphy tube?

19-5. Obtain a syringe, and practice inflating and deflating the cuffs of several ET tubes. How much volume is required to inflate a cuff? Does it vary for different-sized tubes?

19-6. Obtain appropriate equipment, and practice measuring ET tube cuff pressure in an artificial (plastic) trachea.

19-7. Using an intubated artificial trachea and positive pressure ventilation, practice the minimal occluding volume (minimum-seal) technique.

CLINICAL PROBLEM-SOLVING: STUDENT EXERCISES

19-8. While working a night shift at a local hospital, you are called to the room of a patient who just suffered a cardiac arrest. List four methods or devices that may be used to ventilate the patient without intubating. _____

_____

_____

_____

19-9. A patient has an nasopharyngeal airway placed appropriately. Shortly afterward, the patient is found gagging and the airway is not seen. What needs to be done? _____

_____

_____

_____

19-10. In the field, a cardiac arrest victim has an esophageal obturator airway (EOA) inserted and ventilation is begun. On assessment, no breath sounds are found, but the abdomen is distending. What steps should be taken? _____

_____

_____

_____

19-11. An adult patient, whose history is unknown, is newly intubated with an ET tube. Breath sounds are present on the left side of the thorax but not on the right. What might be the cause? _____

_____

_____

_____

19-12. Following a difficult nasal intubation using direct laryngeal visualization, 6 mL of air is used to inflate the ET tube cuff. When attempting to ventilate, a large gas leakage is heard coming from around the tube. Another 6 mL of air is injected into the cuff, but the leak persists. What should be done? _____

_____

_____

_____

19-13. While attempting to intubate a patient, it is discovered that the light does not function on the laryngoscope blade. What may be wrong?

_____

_____

_____

19-14. A newborn needs an emergency intubation. How is the appropriate-sized ET tube, needed for intubation, determined? _____

_____

_____

_____

19-15. An intubated, mechanically ventilated patient has just returned from the operating room. You want to evaluate the appropriateness of the cuff pressure, but a manometer is not available. What can be done until a manometer is located? _____

_____

_____

_____

19-16. An intubated patient on a mechanical ventilator has a large leak around the ET tube cuff, even at an elevated cuff pressure. A radiograph has determined that the tube is positioned properly. Why might this leak be occurring, and is the patient in danger of tracheal damage from the elevated cuff pressure?

_____

_____

_____

RESEARCH PROJECTS: STUDENT EXERCISES

19-17. Design a project to measure the pressure exerted against the tracheal wall by an inflated cuff at different cuff pressures and with different size ET tubes. Compare the pressure measured at the cuff-trachea interface to the pressure measured inside the cuff.

19-18. According to Poiseuille's law, resistance to flow is directly related to the length of a tube and inversely related to a tube's diameter. Design a study to measure back pressure and calculate resistance with various tube lengths and sizes at different flow rates.

ENDOTRACHEAL TUBE AND SUCTION CATHETER SIZE

ETs and suction catheters come in many sizes. ET tubes may have several size markings printed on the tube. The outer diameter (OD) is the external diameter of the tube in millimeters. The inner diameter (ID) is the internal diameter of the tube in millimeters. When stating the size of the tube used to intubate a patient, the ID is the number quoted. This number can also be located on the 15-mm ET adapter used for connection to mechanical ventilator circuits or Briggs' adapters. This allows tube size documentation after intubation, if it was not noted before intubation. Another marking that may be present on the ET tube is the French (Fr) size of the tube. This is the external circumference of the tube in millimeters.

Suction catheters are routinely sized by Fr units. Again, this indicates their external circumference in millimeters. Understanding the relationship between suction catheter Fr sizing and ET tube ID sizing is important for determining the appropriate-sized suction catheter to use for a given ET tube size.

The circumference (C) of a circle is equal to the diameter (D) of the circle times π. The Greek letter π is pronounced "pie" and is equal to 3.14. This is expressed in the following formula:

$$C = D \times \pi$$

If either the C or D is known, the other can be calculated.

Calculation of Appropriate Catheter Size for Endotracheal Suctioning: The ½ Rule

In *Respiratory Care*, it is suggested that suction catheters should not have an external diameter larger than ½ the internal diameter of the ET tube through which it will be inserted, "the ½ rule." This is recommended in an attempt to help decrease some of the hazards associated with ET suctioning. Since suction catheters are sized differently than ET tubes, using the above formula can help in determining proper suction catheter size.

Example

Using the ½ rule, what is the maximum-sized suction catheter recommended for use with a #8 ET tube?

The ID of a #8 tube is 8 mm. One half of this value is 4 mm ($0.5 \times 8 = 4$). This means that the largest suction catheter to be used must not have an external diameter of more than 4 mm. By using the formula $C = \pi \times D$, the appropriate suction catheter size can be determined. (For our calculations, $\pi = 3$.)

$$C = \pi \times D = 3 \times 4 = 12 \text{ or a 12-Fr}$$
$$\text{suction catheter}$$

Thus, a 12-Fr catheter, which has a circumference of 12 mm and an external diameter of 4 mm, is the largest suction catheter to be used with a #8 ET tube.

Once this relationship is understood, a simple calculation to determine the largest suction catheter size to be used with any ET tube is to multiply the ET tube size (ID) times 1.5 ($8 \times 1.5 = 12$) (Figure 19-1).

SUCTION PRESSURE REGULATION

There are many types of suction regulators that can be used to create subambient pressure. Regardless of the device used, it must be regulated and monitored to avoid some of the hazards associated with suctioning. The following subambient pressures are recommended for use with suctioning. For infants, use –60 to –80 mmHg; for children, use –80 to –100 mmHg; and for adults, use –100 to –120 mmHg. There are times when pressures exceeding these parameters will be needed. It is best to use the lowest pressure that is still effective for clearing secretions. Review the conversions to inches of mmHg and cmH_2O, since some suction devices may also be calibrated using these pressure units.

Student Exercises

19-19. List several complications associated with endotracheal suctioning. Generate a second list of methods used to help prevent these complications.

19-20. What are the largest-sized suction catheters recommended for use with the following ET tube sizes?

ET Tube Size		Suction Cather (Fr) (1/2 rule)
a.	10	_____
b.	9	_____
c.	8	_____
d.	7	_____
e.	6	_____
f.	5	_____
g.	4	_____

#8 ET tube

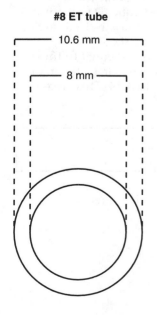

12 Fr suction catheter

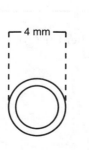

Combination

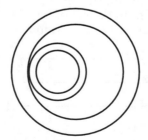

FIGURE 19-1. Illustration of the relationship between a #8 endotracheal (ET) tube and a 12 French (Fr) suction catheter (drawing, 3× actual size).

Laboratory Projects: Student Exercises

19-21. Compare the following vacuum systems: central vacuum, portable suction pump, and venturi suction. Practice making pressure adjustments for different levels of suction pressure required.

19-22. Obtain several types of suction catheters including a curved tip catheter and a closed system suctioning setup. Compare the catheters and demonstrate proper suctioning technique with each.

Research Projects: Student Exercises

19-23. Design a project to measure the amount of volume removed by a suction catheter during suctioning. Set up a known volume of gas (maybe using a water seal spirometer, a plastic bag, or test lung with a known volume of gas). Intubate the container and measure the amount of air removed from it by using different-sized suction catheters, at different suction pressures, for varying amounts of time, and with different-sized ET tubes.

19-24. Design a project to measure the amount of subambient (negative) pressure generated inside a test lung when varying the size of the suction catheter, the size of the ET tube, the suction pressure used, and the time during which the suction is applied.

REVIEW QUESTIONS

19-25. List the three single cartilages that help make up the larynx.

19-26. List the three paired cartilages that help make up the larynx.

19-27. Which of the following is most desirable for a patient who requires periodic mechanical ventilation?
A. a trach button
B. a Jackson metal trach tube
C. an uncuffed plastic trach tube
D. a cuffed fenestrated trach tube

19-28. The turbinates (or conchae) are located where?
A. nasal cavity
B. nasopharynx
C. hypopharynx
D. oropharynx

19-29. When using the straight blade of a laryngoscope, where is the blade tip to be placed?
A. into the trachea
B. into the vallecula, lifting the epiglottis indirectly
C. against the epiglottis, lifting it directly
D. into the oropharyngeal area

19-30. Which plastic is most commonly used for manufacture of ET tubes?
A. teflon
B. polyethylene
C. polyvinylchloride
D. silicon

19-31. The standard laryngoscope and blade is designed to be held in which hand during intubation?
A. the right hand
B. the left hand
C. either hand

19-32. Magill forceps would most likely be used during which of the following procedures?
A. tracheostomy
B. nasotracheal intubation
C. orotracheal intubation
D. extubation

19-33. During normal breathing, the nose and nasopharynx account for what percent of total airway resistance?
A. 20%
B. 30%
C. 40%
D. 50%

19-34. The primary advantage of a fenestrated tracheostomy tube is that it:
A. reduces the incidence of tracheal injury
B. reduces mucus production
C. reduces nosocomial infections
D. facilitates communication

19-35. The vocal cords are protected from external trauma by which cartilage?
A. epiglottis
B. cricoid
C. thyroid
D. cuneiform

19-36. While performing a ventilator check, it is discovered that a small leak around the ET tube cuff occurs during peak pressure of the sigh breath. The cuff is inflated to 20 mmHg.
Which of the following is the most appropriate action to be taken?
A. increase the cuff pressure until the leak stops
B. decrease the cuff pressure to 15 mmHg
C. suggest a larger ET tube be used to replace the present ET tube
D. leave the situation as it is

19-37. Which of the following is not true concerning the trachea?
A. it is 12 to 15 cm long
B. it is 1.8 to 2.5 cm in diameter
C. it is supported by 16 to 22 cartilage rings
D. it is "C" shaped

19-38. While attempting to perform ET suctioning on a patient, the therapist is unable to clear the thick secretions. The ET tube is a #7, the suction catheter is a Fr 14, and the suction pressure is set at –80 mmHg. Which of the following is the most appropriate action to be taken?
   A. obtain a Fr 16 suction catheter
   B. replace the suction regulator
   C. increase the suction pressure to –120 mmHg
   D. attach the suction tubing directly to the ET tube

19-39. The tip of the curved laryngoscope blade is placed into what area?
   A. ventricle
   B. vallecula
   C. vestibule
   D. infraglottic cavity

19-40. Overinflation of the cuff of an ET tube would most likely result in which of the following?
   A. decreased local capillary blood flow
   B. laryngospasm
   C. decreased lung compliance
   D. increased airway resistance

19-41. The most appropriate means to maintain a patent airway in an unconscious patient who is not intubated is to:
   A. sit the patient up
   B. place a pillow under the head
   C. perform the head tilt/chin lift maneuver
   D. place the patient in the prone position

19-42. Which of the following are appropriate for helping to determine proper ET tube placement?

   I. chest radiograph
   II. auscultation of the epigastrium
   III. auscultation of the chest bilaterally
   IV. observing the depth markings on the ET tube

   A. I and III only
   B. I, III, and IV only
   C. I, II, and III only
   D. I, II, III, and IV

19-43. Ideally, tracheal tube cuff pressures should not exceed:
   A. 10 mmHg
   B. 15 mmHg
   C. 20 mmHg
   D. 25 mmHg

19-44. Appropriate suction pressures for adult patients should be in the subambient range of:
   A. 60 to 80 mmHg
   B. 80 to 100 mmHg
   C. 100 to 120 mmHg
   D. 120 to 140 mmHg

19-45. 20 mmHg is equal to approximately how many cmH_2O?
   A. 37
   B. 27
   C. 20
   D. 14

19-46. 100 mmHg is equal to approximately how many inches of Hg?
   A. 2 inHg
   B. 4 inHg
   C. 6 inHg
   D. 8 inHg

19-47. The narrowest part of the adult airway is the opening of which of the following?
   A. cricoid cartilage
   B. false vocal cords
   C. true vocal cords
   D. trachea

19-48. Which size ET tube will result in the greatest work of breathing?
   A. 8.0 mm
   B. 7.5 mm
   C. 7.0 mm
   D. 6.5 mm

19-49. Which of the following is the most appropriate tube insertion length for an average male (measured from the incisors)?
   A. 21 cm
   B. 23 cm
   C. 25 cm
   D. 27 cm

19-50. An adult female orally intubated to a depth of 20 cm is being reintubated nasally. What depth is an appropriate approximation?
   A. 17 cm
   B. 20 cm
   C. 23 cm
   D. 26 cm

19-51. Which of the following is correct for maximum cuff pressure for an ET tube?
   A. 2.7 kPa
   B. 20 cmH_2O
   C. 27 mmHg
   D. 40 cmH_2O

19-52. Which of the following may change the intracuff or cuff-tracheal interface pressure?
   A. use of nitrous oxide
   B. tube movement
   C. leak at pilot balloon
   D. all of the above

19-53. Which of the following laryngoscope blades does not lift the epiglottis directly?
   A. Miller
   B. Wisconsin
   C. McIntosh
   D. Flag

19-54. Which of the following is true concerning an ET tube cuff?
   A. it prevents aspiration
   B. it prevents tube movement
   C. the same size cuff will require different volumes to create a seal in different patients
   D. it will cause no tracheal mucosal damage as long as the pressure in the cuff is below 20 mmHg

20

Mechanical Ventilation of the Adult Patient

STUDENT EXERCISES

20-1. List five indications for mechanical ventilation. (Refer to Table 20-1 in *Respiratory Care*.) _____

_____

_____

20-2. List five factors affecting airway pressure with volume ventilation. (Refer to Table 20-5 in *Respiratory Care*.) _____

_____

_____

_____

20-3. List five factors affecting tidal volume with pressure ventilation. (Refer to Table 20-6 in *Respiratory Care*.) _____

_____

_____

_____

20-4. List three factors affecting mean airway pressure during positive pressure ventilation. (Refer to Table 20-8 in *Respiratory Care*.) _____

_____

_____

20-5. A 175-lb, 48-year-old man is placed on mechanical ventilation with the following settings: f = 12 breaths/min, V_T = 900 mL, Flow = 35 L/min, FIO_2 = 50%:

  a. Calculate the following: T_I ____, T_E ____, I:E ____, and V_E ____.
  b. Arterial blood gases (ABGs) on the above settings reveal the following: pH = 7.51, $PaCO_2$ = 28 mmHg, PaO_2 = 178 mmHg, O_2Sat = 99%, and HCO_3 = 28 mEq/L.

Interpret the ABG results. _____

_____

_____

_____

What changes should be made? _____

_____

_____

_____

Calculate the predicted FIO_2 needed to reduce the PaO_2 to 90 mmHg._____

_____

_____

_____

20-6. A 20-year-old, 105-lb woman presents to the emergency room. She is apneic owing to a drug overdose. She is intubated and transferred to the intensive care unit (ICU) where she is placed on mechanical ventilation. ____

_____

_____

_____

  a. Select appropriate ventilator settings for this patient: f ____ breaths/min, V_T ____ mL, FIO_2 ____ %, and Flow rate ____ L/min.
  b. Twenty minutes after the patient is stabilized on mechanical ventilation (MV), her blood gases reveal the following: pH = 7.54, $PaCO_2$ = 25 mmHg, PaO_2 = 70 mmHg, HCO_3 = 23 mEq/L, O_2Sat = 96%. What specific ventilator changes would you recommend at this time? _____

_____

_____

_____

20-7. A 45-year-old, 198-lb man is brought to the ICU after suffering a cardiac arrest. He is placed on MV with the following settings: f = 8/min, V_T = 800 mL, FIO_2 = 40%, Flow = 40 L/min. ABGs reveal pH = 7.30, $PaCO_2$ = 47 mmHg, PaO_2 = 52 mmHg, O_2Sat = 84%, HCO_3 = 18 mEq/L.

    a. Calculate the following: V_A _____ L, a/A _____, A-a _____ mmHg, I:E _____.
    b. What ventilator changes would you make?

    _____

    _____

    _____

20-8. A 140-lb man presents to the emergency department in severe respiratory distress. The patient has course crackles over the left posterior basilar lung fields. His temperature is 102°F. Chest radiograph shows an infiltrate in the left lower lobe with hyperaeration throughout both lung fields. The patient, who is 55 years old, states that he has smoked three packs a day for the past 40 years. ABGs on 2 L/min reveal pH = 7.26, $PaCO_2$ = 89 mmHg, PaO_2 = 34 mmHg, O_2Sat = 60%, HCO_3 = 36 mEq/L. The decision is made to intubate and ventilate the patient.

    a. Select the following: mode of ventilation _____, f _____ /min, V_T _____ mL, FIO_2 _____ %, Flow _____ L/min.
    b. After stabilization, you determine the patient is air trapping. What changes could you make to help relieve this condition?

    _____

    _____

    _____

    c. Interpret the ABG obtained in the emergency department. _____

    _____

    _____

    _____

    d. What type of pulmonary problem does this patient appear to have?_____

    _____

    _____

    _____

20-9. A 28-year-old, 130-lb woman is admitted to the ICU following an automobile accident with both head and thoracic injuries. The pa-

tient is not breathing and her lung/thorax compliance is low._____

_____

_____

_____

    a. Choose appropriate MV settings. Mode _____, f _____ /min, V_T _____ mL, FIO_2 _____ %, flow _____ L/min.
    b. Thirty minutes into MV, the patient suddenly becomes cyanotic, peak pressure rises significantly, and O_2Sat drops from 97% to 70%. What pulmonary problem might you suspect? How would this problem best be treated? _____

    _____

    _____

20-10. List the minimal mechanical values considered necessary to institute weaning. (Refer to table 20-14 in *Respiratory Care*.) _____

_____

_____

_____

MIP
VC
FEV_1
Resting V_E
Compliance
MVV
Spontaneous V_T
Spontaneous rate
Rate/V_T ratio

REVIEW QUESTIONS

20-11. Which of the following mechanical indicators suggest the need for mechanical ventilation?
    A. respiratory rate 25 to 30/min
    B. minute ventilation 5 to 10 L/min
    C. maximum inspiratory force <−20 cmH_2O
    D. vital capacity >15 mL/Kg

20-12. Which of the following gas exchange indicators suggest the need for mechanical ventilation?
    A. $P(A-a)O_2$ > 200 mmHg on 100% oxygen
    B. PaO_2 < 60 mmHg on an FIO_2 of > 60%
    C. PaO_2/FIO_2 < 400
    D. V_D/V_T > 0.40

20-13. To avoid pressure injury to the lung during mechanical ventilation, alveolar pressure should be maintained less than what pressure?
A. 25 cmH$_2$O
B. 30 cmH$_2$O
C. 35 cmH$_2$O
D. 40 cmH$_2$O

20-14. Mechanically ventilated patients are at increased risk for gastrointestinal bleeding. Which of the following is not a treatment for this condition?
A. natriuretic peptide
B. H$_2$ blockers
C. sucralfate
D. antacids

20-15. Urine output may decrease during mechanical ventilation for each of the following reasons except:
A. decreased cardiac output
B. decreased plasma antidiuretic hormone (ADH) level
C. decreased blood pressure
D. decreased renal perfusion

20-16. Plateau pressures higher than 35 cmH$_2$O may be safe and not cause lung damage if:
A. the V$_T$ is small
B. the lung is very compliant
C. auto-PEEP is < 10 cmH$_2$O
D. the chest wall has a low compliance

20-17. To help prevent oxygen toxicity, the F$_{IO_2}$ should be maintained less than which of the following maximum values?
A. 40%
B. 50%
C. 60%
D. 70%

20-18. Negative intermittent positive pressure ventilation (NIPPV) should not be used in each of the following cases except in:
A. patients with acute exacerbations of chronic respiratory failure
B. patients with large volumes of secretions
C. patients with upper airway obstruction
D. patients at risk for aspiration

20-19. Each of the following statements is true concerning noninvasive ventilation except:
A. it is not always successful
B. it is time consuming
C. mask fit is very important
D. a flow-cycled mode should be used

20-20. A mode of ventilation allowing the patient to determine their own rate and V$_T$, yet helping to decrease the work of breathing (WOB) by augmenting the patient's effort is:
A. control
B. PSV
C. SIMV
D. A/C

20-21. Flow triggering has been shown to be superior to pressure triggering in which of the following modes of ventilation?
A. CPAP
B. PSV
C. SIMV
D. A/C.

20-22. The main disadvantage of volume-limited ventilation is:
A. delivered volumes are not guaranteed
B. inspiratory time is too long
C. high peak alveolar pressures can result
D. flow rates are not adjustable

20-23. Which of the following is the major factor determining whether auto-PEEP will occur?
A. length of T$_I$
B. length of T$_E$
C. flow rate
D. V$_T$

20-24. When comparing inspiratory flow patterns, which seems to be the most desirable?
A. constant flow
B. sine wave flow
C. decelerating flow
D. square wave flow

20-25. An appropriate PEEP level for most patients suffering from ARDS seems to be in the range of:
A. 3 to 5 cmH$_2$O
B. 5 to 8 cmH$_2$O
C. 8 to 12 cmH$_2$O
D. 12 to 15 cmH$_2$O

20-26. Which of the following will increase mean airway pressure?
A. increased peak airway pressure
B. increased respiratory rate
C. increased flow rate
D. all of the above

20-27. Which of the following is true concerning mechanical dead space?
A. it is the same as volume loss caused by compression
B. it is rebreathed gas
C. it significantly decreases the volume of gas reaching the lungs
D. addition of mechanical V$_D$ may cause PaCO$_2$ levels to drop

20-28. Clinical signs of ventilator-patient dyssynchrony may include each of the following except:
A. patient agitation
B. bradypnea
C. chest retractions
D. chest-abdominal paradox

20-29. The best indicator for respiratory muscle fatigue is probably which of the following?
A. tachypnea
B. abdominal paradox
C. increased PaCO$_2$
D. decreased maximum inspiratory pressure (MIP)

20-30. If respiratory muscle fatigue occurs, how long should the patient be rested?
   A. 4 to 8 hours
   B. 8 to 16 hours
   C. 16 to 24 hours
   D. 24 hours or longer

20-31. For an alert and oriented patient, the first thing that should be done for a patient who is going to be weaned is to:
   A. obtain all parameters
   B. switch the patient to a weaning mode
   C. do an ABG
   D. prepare the patient mentally for the weaning plan

20-32. Which of the following is the best indicator for evaluation of tissue hypoxia?
   A. PvO_2
   B. PaO_2
   C. FiO_2
   D. PAO_2

21

Mechanical Ventilation

21-1. List the four phase variables of a mechanical breath.

a. _____

b. _____

c. _____

d. _____

21-2. List the four factors that can trigger (start) a mechanical breath.

a. _____

b. _____

c. _____

d. _____

21-3. Define inspiratory time. _____

_____

_____

_____

21-4. List the four factors that normally cycle (terminate) a mechanical ventilator breath.

a. _____

b. _____

c. _____

d. _____

LABORATORY EXERCISES

For each of the following exercises, select a mechanical ventilator, assemble and connect the appropriate circuit, and attach a test lung to the patient connector.

21-5. Examine the dials, touch pads, and so on, and become familiar with their operation. Turn the ventilator on, and adjust the settings for a normal routine patient situation with normal resistance and compliance. Settings are as follows: A/C, volume (flow) cycled, frequency of 10/min, VT of 800 mL, (VE of 8.0 L) FIO$_2$ of 50%, positive end-expiratory pressure (PEEP) of +4 cmH$_2$O, sensitivity of –1 cmH$_2$O, flow rate (FR) of 50 L/min, and a pressure limit of 60 cmH$_2$O. Set other parameters and alarm limits as appropriate. Document the actual exhaled volume and peak inspiratory pressure (PIP) required to deliver the volume. Create a high-pressure condition and check for proper alarm and termination of breath. Does the ventilator pressure alarm respond to internal machine pressure or proximal system (patient) pressure? Repeat this exercise with several mechanical ventilators.

21-6. While actively generating negative pressure by manipulation of the test lung, test each of the following modes of ventilation: control, A/C, synchronized intermittent mandatory ventilation (SIMV), pressure support, and pressure control. Perform this exercise using different ventilators and at different sensitivity settings. *Personal Note:* The control mode of ventilation, where a patient is unable to initiate a breath, should not be used in patient care. If it is desired that a patient not breathe spontaneously, the patient should be sedated or hyperventilated and hyperoxygenated so they do not assist. If a patient is apneic, there is no need to use the control mode. I think the control mode should be removed from the mode choices on a ventilator panel.

21-7. Select a mechanical ventilator with digital readouts for inspiratory time (TI), PIP, inspiratory to expiratory ratio (I:E), and so on, or obtain an in-line monitor that can measure these parameters. Also obtain a test lung with adjustable resistance and compliance settings. Set up a normal patient situation in the volume-cycled mode with normal resistance (R), compliance (C), and ventilator settings. Document each of the settings: C, R, FR, flow pattern (FP), and VT. Also document each of the resultants: TI, PIP, and I:E. After recording each of these, start by making one change at a time, and document the effect of that change. Evaluate the effects caused by these changes.

Parameter Change	Resultants		
	TI	PIP	I:E
Increase R	____	____	____
Decrease R	____	____	____
Increase C	____	____	____
Decrease C	____	____	____
Increase FR	____	____	____
Decrease FR	____	____	____
Change FP	____	____	____
Change FP	____	____	____
Increase VT	____	____	____
Decrease VT	____	____	____

21-8. Repeat exercise 21-7 with the ventilator in the time-cycled pressure-limited (pressure control) mode. Set up a normal patient situation with normal R, C, and ventilator settings. Document each of the settings: C, R, FR, TI, and PIP. Also document the resultant VT. After documenting each of these, start by making one change at a time, and document the effect of that change. Evaluate the effect caused by these changes.

Parameter Change	Resultant, VT
Increase R	____
Decrease R	____
Increase C	____
Decrease C	____
Increase FR	____
Decrease FR	____
Increase PIP	____
Decrease PIP	____

21-9. If a graphics package is available on the mechanical ventilator being studied, evaluate the flow-volume or pressure-volume curves generated by the parameter changes made in exercises 21-7 and 21-8.

21-10. Set up a "normal" patient on mechanical ventilation. Document the FIO_2 at the patient connector and the delivered VT. Using appropriate equipment, deliver an in-line aerosol treatment by two methods:

1. the ventilator's built-in nebulizer system, if present
2. a small-volume nebulizer (SVN) powered from an external flowmeter.

Document the change in FIO_2 and VT for each of these methods. Does the use of the nebulizer affect the sensitivity of the system? Compare the two methods and list some advantages and disadvantages for each.

Calculating Volume Based on Flow Rate and Time

Many times, delivered volume is displayed by the ventilator, but delivered tidal volume can be determined based on the set flow rate and the inspiratory time using the following formula:

$$Volume = Flow \times Time$$

Where: Volume is the delivered VT in L

Flow is the average flow rate (FR) in L/sec (to change L/min to L/sec, divide L/min by 60)

Time is the inspiratory time in seconds

Student Exercise
Calculate the VT based on the given information.

	Given		Calculate
	FR L/min	TI sec	VT L
21-11.	60	1.0	____
21-12.	40	1.2	____
21-13.	30	0.8	____
21-14.	50	1.5	____
21-15.	80	0.6	____

Be aware that the above formula is not appropriate for calculation of delivered VT during pressure-limited (pressure control) ventilation. This condition is discussed in the following section.

INFANT VENTILATORS

Time-Cycled, Pressure-Limited Ventilation

Usually, infant ventilators are time-cycled, although some are said to have volume-cycling capabilities. Infant ventilation is often carried out by using a pressure-limited mode. This means that a preset pressure limit is reached and held as a pressure plateau for the duration of TI that is time-cycled. Depending on the length of TI, there are several factors that can affect VT in this mode of ventilation. For a short TI, when alveolar pressure (Palv) does not equilibrate with system pressure (Psys), the following may all affect VT: TI, patient airway resistance (Raw), and lung-thorax C (Raw × C equals what is known as a time constant), PIP, and flow rate. For a longer TI, when Palv equilibrates with Psys, only ΔP and compliance will determine VT. ΔP represents the pressure difference between PEEP level and PIP. VT is directly proportional to both C and ΔP. When using this method of ventilation (Palv = Psys), volume loss owing to compression does not "rob" the patient of volume or change the actual patient VT. The actual patient VT can be measured by using a pneumotachometer placed in the dead space of the circuit, that is, attached to the endotracheal tube. VT will vary as compliance changes and VT cannot be calculated unless the patient's compliance is known. The formula for determining C is:

$$C = V/\Delta P$$

where: V is VT and

ΔP is (PIP − PEEP)

Rewritten: V = C × ΔP and if C is known, VT can be calculated

Example
An infant on a ventilator has a lung compliance of 2 mL/cmH$_2$O. His PEEP level is +4 cmH$_2$O and his PIP is 20 cmH$_2$O. What VT is delivered to his lungs?

$$V = C \times \Delta P$$

$$V_T = C \times (PIP - PEEP)$$

$$V_T = 2 \text{ mL/cmH}_2O \times (20 - 4 \text{ cmH}_2O)$$

$$V_T = 2 \times 16 = 32 \text{ mL}$$

Student Exercise
Calculate the VT based on the given information.

	Given		Calculate
	Cst mL/cmH$_2$O	ΔP cmH$_2$O	VT L
21-16.	20	40	_____ adult
21-17.	40	30	_____ adult
21-18.	30	20	_____ adult
21-19.	4	10	_____ infant
21-20.	1	25	_____ infant

Time-Cycled, Volume-Limited Ventilation

Another method of infant ventilation is accomplished by setting a desired flow rate and TI while not pressure limiting. In this case, the delivered VT is determined by TI and FR and can be calculated. However, it will not be the actual volume delivered to the patient. During this method of ventilation, volume loss owing to compression does rob the patient of some of the delivered volume.

Example
An infant is being ventilated by an infant ventilator set at a flow of 6 L/min and with a TI of 0.4 seconds. A pressure limit is not being reached. Calculate the delivered VT.

$$(FR \times T_I)/60 = V_T$$

$$(6 \times 0.4)/60 = V_T$$

$$2.4/60 = V_T$$

$$0.04 \text{ L} = V_T$$

$$0.04 \text{ L} \times 1000 \text{ mL/L} = 40 \text{ mL}$$

Student Exercise
Calculate the VT based on the given information.

	Given		Calculate
	FR L/min	TI, sec	VT, mL
21-21.	15	0.3	_____
21-22.	10	0.6	_____
21-23.	12	0.5	_____
21-24.	8	0.4	_____
21-25.	6	0.6	_____

Although the typical infant circuit will have a compression factor (Cf) lower than its adult counterpart, volume loss caused by compression (VL) can be significant. The actual VT the patient receives can be much less than the volume delivered by the machine during this method of ventilation. In the previous example, if the Cf is 1 mL/cmH$_2$O and the ΔP is 20 cmH$_2$O, the VL is 20 mL (1 × 20). This would account for 50% of the delivered volume.

Because, during volume limited ventilation, a pressure limit is not reached, VT tends to stay a little more consistent even in the face of compliance changes. Also, compliance changes may be followed since increased compliance will result in a lower PIP and decreased compliance will result in an increased PIP. Regardless of the type of ventilation performed, if a leak occurs around the uncuffed tube, volume will be lost and the actual volume may not be the same as the measured or calculated volumes. Note that some infant ventilators do allow the setting of a delivered VT. These machines integrate flow rate and TI to deliver the desired set volume.

Many advances have been made in infant ventilation. These include the use of pneumotachometers, synchronized ventilation, flow-triggering, and airway graphic analysis. Airway graphics aid in the determination of several mechanical and physiologic parameters. These include peak flow, presence of air leak, incomplete exhalation, patient-ventilator synchrony, optimal PEEP levels, pulmonary overdistention, work of breathing, and dynamic compliance. Airway graphic analysis will continue to play an increased role in infant and adult ventilation.

Laboratory Exercise

21-26. Select an infant mechanical ventilator. Assemble the appropriate circuit, and attach a test lung to the patient connector. Examine the dials, touch pads, and so on, and become familiar with their operation. Turn the ventilator on, and adjust the settings for a normal routine patient situation with normal R and C using the following: intermittent mandatory ventilation, time cycled, frequency of 30/min, TI of 0.5 seconds, FIO_2 of 40%, PEEP of +4 cmH_2O, FR of 8 L/min, and a pressure limit of 20 cmH_2O. Set other parameters and alarm limits as appropriate. Create some situations causing alarm responses. Did the alarms respond appropriately?

Repeat this exercise with several mechanical ventilators. Notice that pressure limit adjustment for pressure-limited ventilation is not labeled as "inspiratory pressure level above PEEP" as it is in adult ventilators. Upper pressure limits will not be adjusted upward or downward automatically as PEEP levels are changed, as they are on adult ventilators. They must be manually adjusted, if desired.

REVIEW QUESTIONS

21-27. After changing the circuit on a mechanical ventilator, the respiratory care practitioner (RCP) notes that the volume is registering 300 mL less than before and that the peak pressure is half of what it was. Which of the following could be the source of the problem?
A. the circuit has a hole in the tubing
B. the humidifier is not assembled tightly and a leak is occurring
C. the medication nebulizer is not connected tightly and leaks
D. all of the above

21-28. An infant is being ventilated in a time-cycled, pressure-limited mode. He has a peak pressure of 23 cmH_2O and a mean airway pressure of 12 cmH_2O. The RCP decreases the inspiratory time. Which of the following responses would now be expected?
A. decreased expiratory phase
B. increased peak pressure
C. increased tidal volume
D. decreased mean airway pressure

21-29. An RCP is called to the intensive care unit to check an adult patient who is being mechanically ventilated. Minimum exhaled volume is being recorded, and the pressure alarm is sounding on each inspiration. The first action should be to:
A. call the supervisor
B. increase the pressure limit setting
C. increase the tidal volume setting
D. attempt to manually ventilate the patient

21-30. An adult patient is receiving ventilatory support with volume-cycled ventilation with the following settings. Mode, A/C; FIO_2, 0.40; VT, 800 mL; and frequency, 12/min. The RCP hears the low volume alarm and observes that the system pressure only reaches 7 cmH_2O during the inspiratory phase. Which of the following should be done?
A. reconnect the exhalation valve line
B. increase the pressure limit
C. straighten the kink in the inspiratory line
D. empty the condensate from the circuit

21-31. A neonate is receiving pressure-limited mechanical ventilation. The physician requests an increase in mean airway pressure. Which of the following could be recommended?
A. increase the inspiratory time
B. decrease the pressure limit
C. increase the expiratory time
D. decrease the rate

21-32. While checking a ventilator that has a heated humidifier, it is noted that there is very little water in the tubing and it does not need to be drained. The most likely explanation is that the:
A. ventilator rate is set very low
B. heating element is not functioning properly
C. flow is set too low
D. room temperature is lower than normal

21-33. A mechanical ventilator set to volume cycle is time cycling at a 1:1 ratio. Which of the following could be adjusted to eliminate the time cycling?
A. increase volume
B. increase respiratory rate
C. increase sensitivity
D. increase peak flow rate

21-34. A breathing circuit's compression factor is determined by cycling a known volume into an occluded circuit and dividing it by:
A. peak inspiratory pressure plus baseline pressure
B. peak inspiratory pressure minus baseline pressure
C. baseline pressure
D. end-inspiratory pause pressure plus baseline pressure

21-35. Given the following data for an infant ventilator, calculate the tidal volume: T_I = 0.5 seconds, T_E = 1 second, flow rate = 7 L/min, pressure limit not reached.
A. 1.6 mL
B. 5.8 mL
C. 16 mL
D. 58 mL

21-36. During infant pressure-limited ventilation, V_T is measured at 22 mL, PEEP is +4 cmH_2O, and PIP is 16 cmH_2O. Calculate compliance.
A. 1.4 mL/cmH_2O
B. 1.8 mL/cmH_2O
C. 3.2 mL/cmH_2O
D. 5.5 mL/cmH_2O

21-37. An infant's compliance, while on pressure-limited mechanical ventilation, is measured to be 1 mL/cmH_2O, PIP is 28 cmH_2O, and PEEP is +6 cmH_2O. Calculate the delivered V_T.
A. 17 mL
B. 22 mL
C. 28 mL
D. 34 mL

21-38. During pressure-control ventilation on an infant ventilator, the PIP is increased with no other changes. How will this affect the V_T?
A. increase V_T
B. decrease V_T
C. no change in V_T

21-39. During pressure-limited ventilation on an infant ventilator, the PEEP level is increased with no other changes. How will this affect V_T?
A. increase V_T
B. decrease V_T
C. no change in V_T

21-40. During adult volume-cycled ventilation, increasing the flow rate will result in which of the following?
A. decreased PIP
B. decreased T_I
C. increased V_T
D. increased frequency

21-41. During adult volume-cycled ventilation, decreasing the V_T will result in which of the following?
A. increased T_I
B. decreased PIP
C. increased compliance
D. decreased T_E

21-42. Delivery of an aerosol treatment, during mechanical ventilation, with a SVN powered by a wall flowmeter, will result in which of the following?
A. decreased sensitivity
B. increased PIP
C. increased V_T
D. all of the above

22

Cardiopulmonary Resuscitation

It is imperative that health care providers be trained in basic life support. It is highly recommended that respiratory care practitioners (RCPs), including students, be certified in advanced cardiac life support (ACLS) as well. Chapter 22 in *Respiratory Care* discusses much information pertinent to both BLS and ACLS training.

VENTILATORY ASSISTANCE

There are many types of devices used for ventilatory assistance during resuscitation. The bag-valve (B-V) or bag-valve-mask (B-V-M) units are popular adjuncts for performing rescue breathing. In many cases, the use of resuscitation devices allows appropriate volume delivery at an appropriate respiratory rate while incorporating delivery of supplemental O_2. Other devices used for ventilatory assistance include mouth-to-mask units and face shields. These devices are often not used because of fear of cross-contamination of infectious agents.

Laboratory Exercises

Listed below are a few suggestions for studies that are easy to perform and will increase your knowledge of resuscitation devices. All three types of units—adult, pediatric, and infant—should be evaluated.

22-1. *Volume delivery:* Using a resuscitator bag, a volume-measuring device that can be attached to the bag, and a test lung, mea-

sure the volumes that can be delivered under varying conditions, such as:

one hand squeezing the bag with nothing attached

two hands squeezing the bag with nothing attached

test lung with a low compliance and normal resistance

test lung with a high compliance and normal resistance

test lung with a low resistance and normal compliance

test lung with a high resistance and normal compliance

This exercise can be repeated for several different bags. Chart all results for comparison. The total volume of each bag should be known. This can be found by looking in the product literature or by filling the bag with water and measuring the volume. Also, attempt to squeeze out all the air possible from the bag. How does this volume compare with the total bag volume? How does it compare with the volumes achieved in the exercise above?

22-2. *Volume delivery:* Using a mannequin for rescue breathing, measure the actual volume delivered under various conditions with different devices:

using different face shields

using different mouth-to-mask devices

using different B-V-M units with one person and two persons manipulating the bag, mask, and airway

22-3. *FiO₂ delivery:* Using various B-V units and an O_2 analyzer, determine the FiO_2 delivered by these devices under varying conditions. These may include the following:

changing the O_2 flow rate

changing the tidal volume (stroke volume) delivered from the unit

changing the rate of ventilation

use of a reservoir that varies in size

manually restricting the recoil of the bag, thus increasing the time allowed for the resuscitator bag to fill with gas

Chart the results for each of the trials. What is the most important variable for determining oxygen delivery? Do bags differ in their ability to deliver high oxygen concentrations?

22-4. *Pressure release or pop-off setting:* Using various B-V devices, a test lung, and a pressure-measuring device adapted into the system, measure the pressure at which the pop-off opens, releasing excess pressure into the atmosphere. Compare it with the manufacturer's stated setting. Can the pressure release be over-ridden if desired?

22-5. *Ventilatory rate:* Using different B-V units and a test lung, attempt to ventilate the test lung at different rates. What is the maximum rate at which the device could be used?

22-6. Select a variety of B-V devices. Dismantle each one, and inspect the inlet valve for method of operation. Inspect the patient valve connector for operation during inspiration and exhalation. Reassemble the units. This procedure is very important so that troubleshooting can be done if a bag malfunctions while in use and no other units are available.

THE HEART'S ELECTRICAL SYSTEM AND ELECTROCARDIOGRAM

The following discussion is meant to provide very basic information about the heart, its conduction system, and electrocardiogram (ECG) interpretation. For more information and greater depth of discussion, please refer to a text on cardiology.

The sinoatrial (S-A) node is located in the right atrium at the superior vena cava. It is normally the pacemaker of the heart, since its ability to elicit spontaneous impulses (automaticity), that is, depolarize, occurs more rapidly than in other areas of the heart. Although the depolarization wave will travel over the entire right and left atria, special conduction fibers (internodal pathways) connect the S-A node and A-V node. A special fiber, Bachmann's Bundle, also runs from the S-A node to the left atrium.

The atrioventricular (A-V) node is located in the inferior right atrium above the tricuspid valve. The Bundle of His is a continuation of the A-V node into the ventricular septum. Normally the A-V node/Bundle of His is considered to be the only electrical pathway from the atria to the ventricles, and it allows only one-way passage of current.

The Bundle Branches are the continuation of the electrical system in the ventricular septum and into the ventricular walls. The terminal ends of the Bundle Branches are the Purkinje Fibers. They infiltrate the myocardial muscle fibers (functional syncytium), which allows impulses to travel over the entire heart muscle (Figure 22-1).

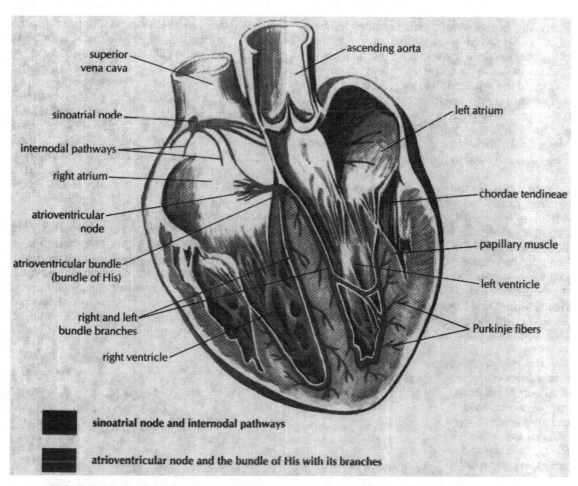

superior vena cava

ascending aorta

sinoatrial node

left atrium

internodal pathways

right atrium

atrioventricular node

chordae tendineae

papillary muscle

atrioventricular bundle (bundle of His)

left ventricle

right and left bundle branches

Purkinje fibers

right ventricle

sinoatrial node and internodal pathways

atrioventricular node and the bundle of His with its branches

FIGURE 22-1. Conduction system. Diagram shows relationships of the sinoatrial node, the atrioventricular node, the common atrioventricular bundle, and its branches.

Normally, each time the S-A node fires, a heartbeat will occur. Actual heart rate can be affected by many factors, such as blood pressure, oxygen demand, body position, exercise, fever, and intrathoracic and intracranial pressure. Stimulation of the sympathetic nervous system will cause heart rate to increase. Stimulation of the parasympathetic nervous system will cause heart rate to decrease.

The ECG is a recording, on the body surface, of the electrical potentials produced by the heart during the cardiac cycle. The ECG paper moves at a speed of 25 mm/sec. Each little block on the paper (1 mm) represents 0.04 sec. Five little blocks equal 0.2 sec. Five larger blocks equal 1.0 sec (Figure 22-2).

The "P" wave is a picture of atrial depolarization. It is normally a positive deflection (rises above the base line or isoelectric line). If the "P" wave is missing, it often indicates that the beat did not originate in the atria but originated in the A-V node/Bundle of His area (junctional beat). The QRS is a picture of ventricular depolarization. The "Q" wave (often not present) is the first negative deflection not preceded by an "R" wave. The "R" wave is the first positive deflection. The "S" wave is the first negative deflection following the "R" wave. Normally, atrial and ventricular contraction will follow the depolarization of the muscle fibers. Since it does, atrial and ventricular rate can be determined by counting the number of "P" waves and QRS complexes. The "T" wave indicates ventricular repolarization and is usually positive. (Each of the above are illustrated in Figure 22-3.) The actual direction of each wave can be influenced by cardiac abnormalities and the leads used to assess the ECG. Although the atria also repolarize, a repolarization wave is not usually seen and would routinely be lost in the QRS complex.

The P-R interval is the time it takes an impulse to travel from the S-A node through the A-V node and Bundle of His, until ventricular depolarization begins. It is measured from the beginning of the "P" wave until the beginning of the QRS complex. (The beginning and ending of waves are determined by their deviation away from the baseline or isoelectric line.) The P-R interval is normally 0.12 to 0.2 seconds long (3 to 5 little blocks). If the P-R interval is increased, there is a conduction delay in the impulse transmission. If the P-R interval is changing, impulses may be occurring in sites other than the S-A node (atrial premature beats), the impulse delay is varying from beat to beat (second degree heart blocks), or the atria and ventricles are beating at their own rates and there is no association between the two complexes (third-degree heart block).

The QRS complex is measured from the beginning of the complex to the end of the complex. It is normally not more than 0.12 seconds long (3 little blocks). The QRS complex will appear normal if the beat originates as an atrial or junctional beat. Beats originating in the ventricles will appear wide and bizarre or "funny looking."

The ST segment is measured from the end of the QRS complex to the beginning of the "T" wave (see Figure 22-3). The ST segment may deviate from baseline for several reasons including, but not limited to, electrolyte imbalance, cardiac ischemia, a myocardial infarction, and pericarditis.

The "R to R" interval can be easily measured from the peak of one "R" wave to the peak of the next "R" wave. The length of the R-R interval will vary depending on the heart rate. One way to count heart rate in a *regular rhythm* is to measure the R-R interval. If the interval is 0.2 sec (5 little spaces), the heart rate is

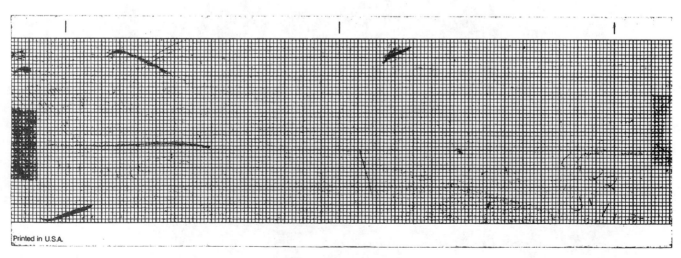

FIGURE 22-2. ECG paper.

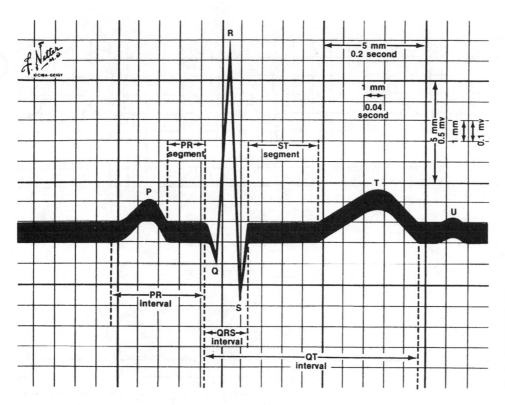

FIGURE 22-3. Electrocardiographic waves, intervals, and segments. (Scheidt S, Erlebacher JA: *Basic Electrocardiography,* p. 15. West Caldwell, NJ. 1986 Ciba-Geigy Corporation. Reproduced with permission.)

300/min; 0.4 seconds (10 little spaces), 150/min; 0.6 sec, (15 spaces), 100/min; and so on. This can be mathematically determined by dividing the length of the R-R interval into 60.

$$60/0.2 = 300; \quad 60/0.6 = 100; \quad 60/0.32 = 187$$

Student Exercise:
Heart Rate Determination

22-7. Determine the heart rate based on the following R-R intervals. Remember this method can only be used for regular rhythms (R-R interval does not change).

R-R Interval (seconds)	Heart Rate (ventricular beats/min)
a. 0.28	_____
b. 0.36	_____
c. 0.48	_____
d. 0.68	_____
e. 0.80	_____
f. 0.96	_____
g. 1.04	_____
h. 1.16	_____
i. 1.32	_____

A second method to determine heart rate in *regular or irregular* (R-R interval constantly changes) rhythms is to count the number of beats (complexes) in a 6-second period and multiply by 10.

Student Exercise:
Cardiac Rhythm Interpretation

For the following cardiac rhythms, determine the following:

Is a "P" wave present? Is it normal? What is the atrial rate?

Is a QRS complex present and normal? What is the ventricular rate?

What relation does the "P" have with the QRS?

Measure the P-R interval.

Interpret the rhythm.

22-8.

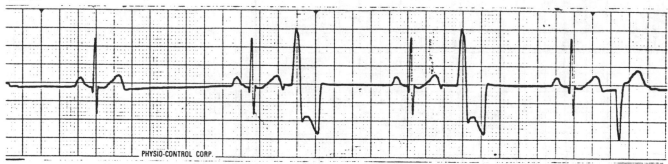

"P" present ____; normal ____; rate ____
"QRS" present ____; normal ____; rate ____
Are the "P" and "QRS" related ____
Length of "P-R" interval ____
Interpretation:_____

22-9.

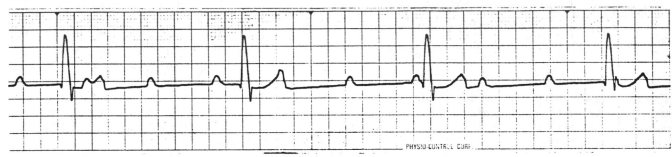

"P" present ____; normal ____; rate ____
"QRS" present ____; normal ____; rate ____
Are the "P" and "QRS" related ____
Length of "P-R" interval ____
Interpretation:_____

22-10.

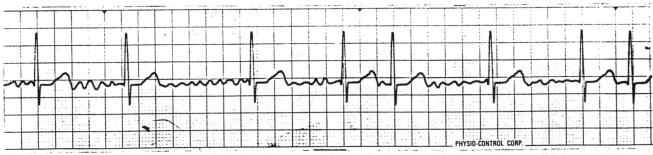

"P" present ____; normal ____; rate ____
"QRS" present ____; normal ____; rate ____
Are the "P" and "QRS" related ____
Length of "P-R" interval ____
Interpretation:_____

22-11.

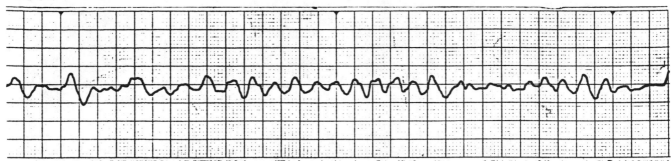

"P" present ____; normal ____; rate ____
"QRS" present ____; normal ____; rate ____
Are the "P" and "QRS" related ____
Length of "P-R" interval ____
Interpretation:_____

22-12.

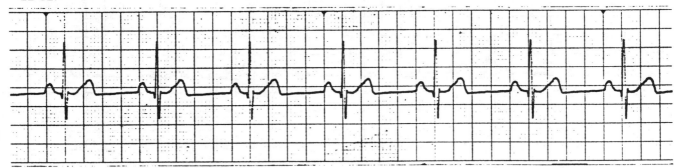

"P" present ____; normal ____; rate ____
"QRS" present ____; normal ____; rate ____
Are the "P" and "QRS" related ____
Length of "P-R" interval ____
Interpretation:_____

22-13.

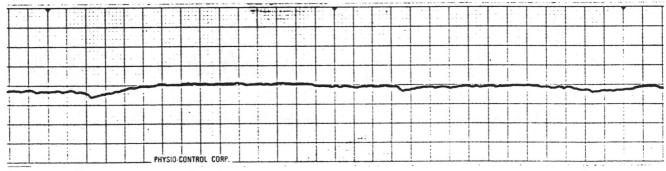

"P" present ____; normal ____; rate ____
"QRS" present ____; normal ____; rate --
Arc the "P" and "QRS" related ____
Length of "P-R" interval ____
Interpretation:_____

22-14.

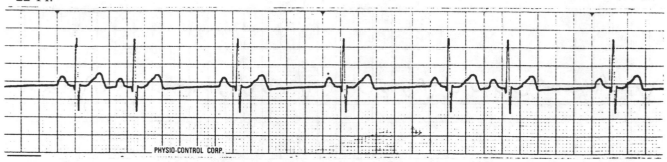

"P" present ____; normal ____; rate ____
"QRS" present ____; normal ____; rate ____
Are the "P" and "QRS" related ____
Length of "P-R" interval ____
Interpretation:_____

22-15.

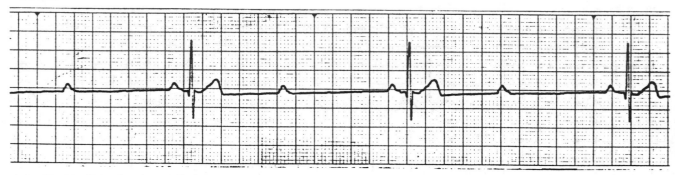

"P" present ____; normal ____; rate ____
"QRS" present ____; normal ____; rate ____
Are the "P" and "QRS" related ____
Length of "P-R" interval ____
Interpretation:_____

22-16.

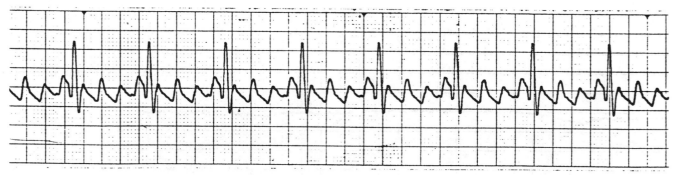

"P" present ____; normal ____; rate ____
"QRS" present ____; normal ____; rate ____
Are the "P" and "QRS" related ____
Length of "P-R" interval ____
Interpretation:_____

22-17.

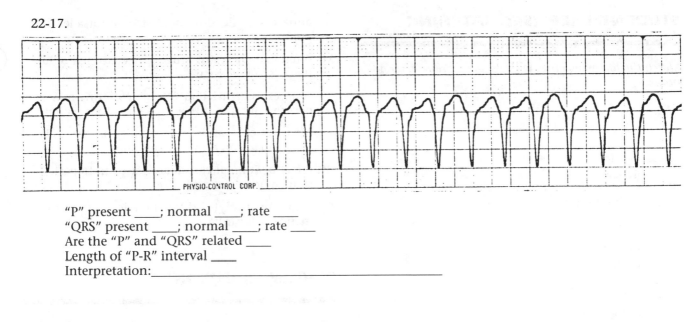

PHYSIO-CONTROL CORP.

"P" present ____; normal ____; rate ____
"QRS" present ____; normal ____; rate ____
Are the "P" and "QRS" related ____
Length of "P-R" interval ____
Interpretation:_____

22-18.

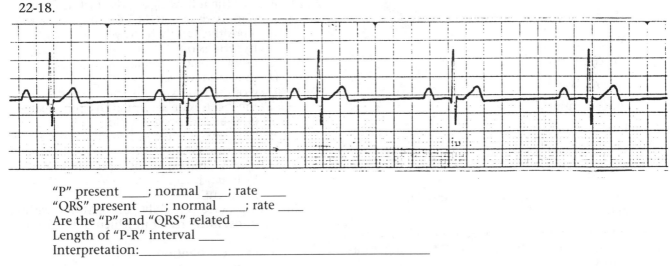

"P" present ____; normal ____; rate ____
"QRS" present ____; normal ____; rate ____
Are the "P" and "QRS" related ____
Length of "P-R" interval ____
Interpretation:_____

22-19.

|————————————— 6 seconds —————————————|

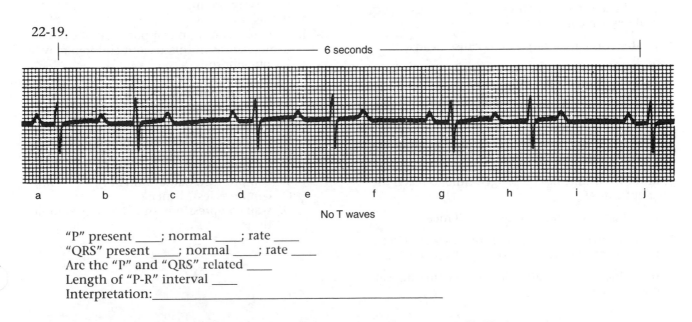

a   b   c   d   e   f   g   h   i   j

No T waves

"P" present ____; normal ____; rate ____
"QRS" present ____; normal ____; rate ____
Are the "P" and "QRS" related ____
Length of "P-R" interval ____
Interpretation:_____

STUDENT EXERCISE: MATCHING

Match the following drugs with the appropriate description.

22-20.

_____ Adenosine

_____ Atropine

_____ Bretylium

_____ Dobutamine

_____ Dopamine

_____ Epinephrine

_____ Lasix

_____ Isuprel

_____ Lidocaine

_____ Magnesium

_____ Morphine

_____ Nitroglycerine

_____ Nitroprusside

_____ Procainamide

_____ Propranolol

_____ Sodium Bicarbonate

_____ Verapamil

A. calcium channel blocker, can be lethal if given in V-tach

B. used to treat pulmonary congestion and congestive heart failure (CHF), dose of 20 to 40 mg intravenously

C. pure beta-adrenergic stimulator, increases myocardial oxygen consumption

D. dilates coronary arteries, may cause headache

E. useful in preexisting hyperkalemia, may be harmful in hypoxic lactic acidosis

F. first drug of choice in pulseless rhythms, do not mix with sodium bicarbonate

G. slows conduction in A-V node, may result in brief asystole after rapid infusion

H. antiarrhythmic, has prolonged time to reach therapeutic dose

I. analgesic, increases venous capacitance

J. dose related to renal, cardiac, or vascular effects; first choice of drugs for moderate hypotension

K. beta blocker, attenuates effects of circulating catecholamines

L. antiarrhythmic, drug of choice for torsades de pointes

M. often first choice of drug for decreasing excitability of ischemic tissue

N. suppresses ventricular ectopy, vomiting may occur with rapid infusion in conscious patient

O. increases myocardial contractility, improves left ventricular function in septic shock

P. direct peripheral vasodilator, used in hypertension emergencies and CHF

Q. parasympatholytic, drug of choice in symptomatic bradycardia

REVIEW QUESTIONS

22-21. Each of the following are risk factors for coronary artery disease (CAD) except:
A. a positive family history
B. hypertension
C. premenopausal female
D. increased stress

22-22. Each of the following are true except:
A. the most frequent initial rhythm in sudden cardiac arrest is V-fib
B. the only effective treatment for V-fib is electrical defibrillation
C. with V-fib the patient is pulseless
D. V-fib tends to convert to V-tach without intervention

22-23. Giving a breath rapidly during M-M breathing will most likely result in which of the following?
A. gastric distention
B. large tidal volumes
C. airway trauma
D. decreased FIO_2

22-24. The most common complication of cardiac compressions in infants and children may be:
A. pneumothorax
B. broken ribs
C. liver laceration
D. bronchial tear

22-25. During appropriate cardiopulmonary resuscitation on an adult, ribs are cracked. Which of the following is most appropriate?
A. compress deeper, 3 inches
B. compress the same, 2 inches
C. compress less, 1 inch
D. stop compressions and give only ventilations

22-26. The most effective method for clearing a partially obstructed airway is:
   A. back blows
   B. chest thrusts
   C. abdominal thrusts
   D. a normal cough

22-27. A conscious obstructive airway victim goes unconscious and is lowered to the floor. The next airway maneuver is:
   A. finger sweep
   B. abdominal thrusts
   C. two breaths
   D. back blows

22-28. With infants, emergency medical service is activated after:
   A. check of responsiveness
   B. two breaths are given
   C. the pulse check
   D. 1 minute of BLS

22-29. Use of the curved laryngoscope blade has each of the following advantages except:
   A. decreased potential for laryngospasm
   B. greater exposure of the glottic opening
   C. conforms to the shape of the tongue
   D. better able to sweep the tongue to the side

22-30. The group responsible for recommending endotracheal tube standards is:
   A. American Society for Testing and Materials (ASTM)
   B. American National Standards Institute (ANSI)
   C. Occupational Safety and Health Administration (OSHA)
   D. Emergency Care Research Institute (ECRI)

22-31. Which of the following, printed on the side of an ET tube, indicates the manufacturer has determined the material is nontoxic by approved methods?
   A. ID
   B. IT
   C. Z-79
   D. F-29

22-32. The name of the technique used to place pressure on the cricoid to help prevent regurgitation during intubation is called the:
   A. Muller maneuver
   B. Sellick maneuver
   C. Valsalva maneuver
   D. Heimlich maneuver

22-33. The suggested volume to be delivered to an adult during M-M breathing is which of the following?
   A. 500 to 700 mL
   B. 600 to 900 mL
   C. 700 to 1000 mL
   D. 800 to 1200 mL

22-34. ASTM and International Organization for Standardization (IOS) have recommended that manual resuscitators be able to deliver a minimum tidal volume and FIO_2 of what amount?
   A. 600 mL and 85%
   B. 700 mL and 90%
   C. 800 mL and 95%
   D. 900 mL and 100%

22-35. ISO standards specify that pressure during B-V ventilation should not exceed:
   A. 35 cmH$_2$O
   B. 40 cmH$_2$O
   C. 45 cmH$_2$O
   D. 50 cmH$_2$O

22-36. For ET tube instillation of medications, it is recommended that what amount of drug be given, diluted with 10 mL of saline or water?
   A. one half of the normal peripheral dose
   B. the same as the normal peripheral dose
   C. two times the normal peripheral dose
   D. four times the normal peripheral dose

22-37. The "P" wave on an ECG strip represents:
   A. atrial depolarization
   B. atrial contraction
   C. ventricular depolarization
   D. ventricular contraction

23

Pulmonary Rehabilitation

STUDENT EXERCISES

23-1. Define pulmonary rehabilitation (PR) in your own words. _____

_____

_____

_____

23-2. List five essential components of a PR program.

a. _____

b. _____

c. _____

d. _____

e. _____

23-3. List five contraindications for a patient being considered for PR.

a. _____

b. _____

c. _____

d. _____

e. _____

CASE STUDY

L. H. is a 55-year-old man who had recently been hospitalized for congestive heart failure (CHF), respiratory insufficiency, and severe chronic obstructive pulmonary disease (COPD). His home medications include metered dose inhalers; Proventil, Atrovent, and Vanceril. He is also on oxygen via nasal cannula at 1 L/min when resting and 3 L/min during exercise.

L. H. presents as a thin male, 121 lb, who is in no acute distress. He has diminished but normal breath sounds, and otherwise has an unremarkable physical examination. His work history includes part-time employment in a furniture store, a paper mill, and work as a bartender. He has had full-time employment as a teacher for 33 years. His father was a heavy smoker and died of lung problems. L. H. has a 45 pack/year smoking history, but stopped smoking several years ago. He reports a history of whooping cough, bronchitis, and pneumonia. He has a chronic cough with expectoration of a small amount of mucoid sputum. He complains of increased shortness of breath (SOB) over the past 10 years, which is aggravated by high humidity and high pollen counts. He has no trouble sleeping and uses only one pillow.

After a thorough evaluation, it was recommended that L. H. be admitted to the pulmonary rehabilitation program. At the beginning of the program, the following tests were conducted:

Pulmonary function tests (PFTs): forced vital capacity (FVC) = 2.58 L (71% pred), forced expiratory volume in 1 second (FEV_1) = 0.44 L (15% pred), bronchodilator produced a significant increase in FVC but no change in flow rates.

Arterial blood gas (ABG): pH = 7.34, $PaCO_2$ = 53 mmHg, HCO_3 = 28 mM/L, PaO_2 = 55 mmHg, and O_2Sat = 87% (room air at rest). With 1 L/min nasal cannula, O_2Sat increased to 90% at rest. With exercise, 6 L/min was required to maintain an O_2Sat at 88%. Following a 6-minute exercise test to determine walking distance, an exercise prescription of biking at 9 mph for 6 minutes or walking for 8 minutes was initiated.

Over the next 6 weeks, the patient was instructed in each of the following areas, and exercise levels were increased as tolerated.

respiratory anatomy and physiology
pursed lip and diaphragmatic breathing
range of motion exercises
signs of overexertion
relaxation techniques
signs of respiratory infections
stair climbing
work simplification
energy conservation
sexual intercourse

cold weather precautions

medication usage

septic techniques

nutrition and hydration

leisure time activities

postural drainage and percussion and coughing

support group availability

At the end of the program, the patient was again formally re-evaluated for progress.

PFT: no change

ABG: pH = 7.35, $PaCO_2$ = 55 mmHg, HCO_3 = 31 mM/L, PaO_2 = 58 mmHg, O_2Sat = 88% (room air at rest). O_2Sat increased to 93% on 1 L/min. With exercise, 3 L/min was required to maintain an O_2Sat of 89%.

By the end of the program, L. H. was biking at 10 mph for 17 minutes or walking for 15 minutes. The patient felt the program was a success. Subjectively he felt better and experiences less shortness of breath. Objectively, he understands his disease process better (post examination) and demonstrated a 31% increase in his exercise tolerance (6-minute walk test).

REVIEW QUESTIONS

23-4. All of the following are true except:
A. lung disease is the leading cause of disability in the United States.
B. only the elderly should be considered for rehabilitation
C. lung disease is the fourth leading cause of mortality in the United States.
D. the course of disease (COPD) can be altered with PR

23-5. Which of the following is correct?
A. all members of the PR team must be involved with the patient
B. patient exercise alone constitutes a PR program
C. a PR program must be individualized
D. the PR program does not need to follow a logical sequence

23-6. To achieve success in a PR program, the patient must have which of the following?
A. a thorough understanding of his or her lung disease
B. behavioral changes to become an active participant
C. an opportunity to use his or her own learning style
D. all of the above

23-7. The most common form of exercise selected for PR is:
A. weight training
B. riding bike
C. swimming
D. walking

23-8. A target heart rate for determining intensity of exercise can be calculated by using which of the following?
A. the Borg scale
B. Karvoner's formula
C. the Bruce protocol
D. the Fagerstrom scale

23-9. All of the following are true except:
A. a patient who exercises at a higher intensity level will not achieve a higher level of fitness
B. duration of exercise should last at least 20 to 30 minutes
C. patients should exercise at least 3 to 4 times a week
D. supplemental oxygen should be given to keep SaO_2 > 90% during exercise

23-10. All of the following are true except:
A. it is important to demonstrate improved status to justify a PR program
B. PR has been shown to reduce the number of days of hospitalization for patients with COPD
C. PR has increased patient ability to carry out activities of daily living
D. almost all studies have shown increased survival in PR patients

23-11. All of the following are true concerning the withdrawal of nicotine except:
A. metabolic rate decreases after nicotine is withdrawn
B. caffeine concentration increases if consumption remains constant
C. theophylline dose needs to be increased by 1/4 to 1/3
D. weight gain is common

23-12. A nicotine "fix" or "hit" occurs:
A. after smoking several cigarettes
B. after smoking one cigarette
C. only with chain smoking
D. 8 seconds after one puff on a cigarette

23-13. The chance of quitting smoking is directly proportional to each of the following except:
A. number of cigarettes smoked
B. education level
C. age (> 50 years)
D. socioeconomic class

23-14. Which of the following has demonstrated the highest success rate of smoking cessation?
A. adverse conditioning
B. group-counseling programs
C. use of special filters
D. acupuncture

23-15. Which of the following has been identified as a "key element to success" for smoking cessation?
A. tapering cigarette use
B. using low-nicotine cigarettes
C. physician's advice to stop
D. setting a firm quitting date and stopping "cold turkey"

24

Respiratory Care in the Home and Alternate Sites

CASE STUDY

G. B. is an 82-year-old man who had been admitted to the hospital with acute respiratory distress. He has a long-standing history of atrial fibrillation, chronic obstructive pulmonary disease (COPD), and pulmonary fibrosis. Before discharge from the hospital, a room air blood gas was drawn and revealed the following.

pH = 7.38, $PaCO_2$ = 48 mmHg, HCO_3 = 28 mM/L, PaO_2 = 54 mmHg, O_2Sat = 89%

G. B. was placed on 1 L/min nasal cannula and an arterial blood gas (ABG) test was repeated.

pH = 7.36, $PaCO_2$ = 48 mmHg, HCO_3 = 27 mM/L, PaO_2 = 87 mmHg, O_2Sat = 96%

After careful consideration of the patient's needs, he and his family were instructed in the use of a portable liquid oxygen system while in the hospital. G. B. was then discharged on 1 L/min. In conjunction with the patient's discharge, a stationary liquid oxygen system was set up at the patient's home by a local home health care

company, of the patient's choosing, and appropriate in-service given.

As it turned out, G. B. improved with time, and more recent ABG analysis revealed an improved PaO_2 (68 mmHg) on room air and with exercise. Home oxygen was able to be discontinued.

REVIEW QUESTIONS

24-1. The primary advantage of a liquid oxygen system is:
   A. greater degree of portability for patients
   B. decreased patient maintenance required
   C. decreased home company visits required
   D. increased ease of use

24-2. The most appropriate oxygen delivery system for a patient is:
   A. tanks and cylinders
   B. a liquid system
   C. an oxygen concentrator
   D. the one that best suits their need

24-3. Medicare guidelines allow for payment of home oxygen for a routine patient if:
   A. PaO_2 < 55 mmHg
   B. PaO_2 < 60 mmHg
   C. SaO_2 < 90%
   D. SaO_2 < 95%

24-4. Each of the following is classified as an oxygen-conserving device except:
   A. transtracheal oxygen delivery systems
   B. reservoir cannula
   C. air-entrainment masks
   D. pulse-oxygen systems

24-5. All of the following are correct concerning home care except:
   A. results in increased cost-effectiveness
   B. results in increased risk of nosocomial infections
   C. improves mental health and social independence
   D. results in decreased rehospitalizations and emergency department visits

24-6. Who is responsible for leading the home care team?
   A. family member
   B. nurse
   C. respiratory care practitioner
   D. doctor

24-7. The primary function of the respiratory care practitioner in home care is to:
   A. provide patient education
   B. instruct patients on use of medical equipment
   C. deliver respiratory therapy treatments
   D. act as a resource person

24-8. The discharge plan should establish each of the following except:
   A. the home care company to supply the services
   B. the treatment plan
   C. the required equipment
   D. advanced directives

24-9. The nocturnal oxygen therapy trial study results demonstrated all of the following except:
   A. decreased mortality rates
   B. improved quality of life
   C. increased exercise tolerance
   D. decreased need for supplemental oxygen

24-10. Which of the following need to be considered for candidacy of mechanical ventilation at home?
   A. family's desires
   B. financial resources
   C. medical stability
   D. all of the above

24-11. Each of the following is correct concerning HMV except:
   A. all caregivers must be able to manage the care of the patient before the patient can go home
   B. a backup ventilator is recommended for patients using HMV for life support
   C. the home ventilator should be as sophisticated as a common hospital ventilator
   D. the home ventilator should be used while the patient is still in the hospital

SECTION V

APPLICATION OF RESPIRATORY CARE TECHNIQUES

25

Neonatal Lung Disease and Respiratory Care

The study of fetal development and the care of newborn infants is one of the most exciting areas in medicine. Experiencing the miracle of birth should bring a never-ending joy. Considering the multitude of problems that could be present, I am always amazed that the majority of births occur without complication. On the other hand, when problems do arise, the scene can become one of sadness and stress in the delivery room or neonatal intensive care unit (NICU). This chapter reviews some of the normal and abnormal situations that present in the fetus and newborn.

FETAL DEVELOPMENT

The following chart lists the developmental event and the approximate gestational time of occurrence associated with it for the average fetus. Please remember that fetal development is not a list of isolated events but a continual dynamic process.

Time of Occurrence	Developmental Event
Day 0	Fertilization in the fallopian tube, usually within 24 hours following ovulation. The fertilized egg (zygote) contains 46 chromosomes.
Day 1	2 cell division (blastomeres)
Day 3	16 cell division (morula)
Days 5–7	The pre-embryonic mass of cells (blastocyst) implants in the uterine wall. Cells begin to differenti-

ate into three distinct layers: ectoderm, mesoderm, and entoderm or endoderm.

Day 14	Now called an embryo (swelling)
Day 20	Diaphragm development begins; head and tail folds appear
Day 22	Primitive heart contracts
Day 24	Lung bud appears as an outpouching of the gut tissue.
Week 4	Embryo is 6-mm long; lens of eye forming; limb buds appear; brain development has begun; lung bud has two branches; nasal cavities forming; tongue development begins; phrenic nerve originates; pulmonary artery and vein develop; placental circulation well developed. The placenta is a highly vascularized area that is responsible for hormone secretion, fetal respiration, and transfer of such things as nutrients, waste products, and antibodies. Although maternal and fetal blood flows are in close contact, these two circulations are separate and *do not* mix.
Week 5	Nostril formation; fingers forming
Week 6	Formation of eyelids, ears and mouth; segmental bronchi present; end of the embryonic period of lung development*
Week 7	Embryo is 25-mm long (1 inch); cartilage rings in trachea; smooth muscle cells of bronchi develop
Week 8	Now called a fetus (young one) and looks human; diaphragm is formed, separating thorax and abdomen; heart is fully formed; formation of teeth in gums; the immune system begins development
Week 9	The head makes up one half the size of the fetus; eyelids fuse; external genitalia differentiating; can see heart beating on sonagram and hear it with use of a sound amplifying device; fetus may suck thumb
Week 10	Vocal cords developing; epithelium consists of superficial layers of columnar cells with cilia development
Week 11	Cartilage in lobar bronchi; kidneys producing urine
Week 12	7.5–8.5 cm long; weighs 1 ounce (28 g); can swallow; basement membrane complete; primitive mucus glands appear with mucus-secreting cells; lung lobes are demarcated; fingernails appear

*Lung development time periods will vary slightly in time of onset and completion from author to author. Terminology may also vary slightly. The stages listed here are as described in *Respiratory Care*.

Week 13	Cilia extent throughout the conducting airways; goblet cells appear
Week 15	Deposition of brown fat begins; breakdown of brown fat is important for heat production following birth
Week 16	Length = 14 cm, weight = 4 ounces (112 g); quickening occurs (mother can feel fetal movements); lanugo (hair) covers the fetal body; the number of conducting airways present will remain relatively unchanged through life; end of the pseudoglandular period of lung development*
Week 18	Vernix caseosa forms (oily substance to protect skin)
Week 20	Lymphatics appear; eyebrows and fingernails well developed; toenails developing; can hear fetal heart beat with the use of a stethoscope on the mother's abdomen
Weeks 22–26	The number of airways with cartilage will remain constant for life; serous cells appear in mucus cells; formation of saccules (primitive alveoli) with type I (squamous pneumocytes) and type II (granular pneumocytes—surfactant producing) alveolar cells; formation of the acinus (the respiratory exchange unit of the lung); the lungs are now developed well enough that life outside the uterus is possible. *This is the earliest time possible for extrauterine life* (at least with today's technology).
Week 26	Eyelids can be opened; brain develops its folds
Week 27	Deposition of non-brown fat begins
Week 28	Carotid chemoreceptors are maturing; end of the canalicular period of lung development*
Week 30	True alveoli may be present
Week 34	The suck/swallow pattern is well developed and effective esophageal peristalsis is present
Weeks 35–36	Lanugo hair is shed; the kidneys, functional at an earlier time, may now pass as much as 500 mL of urine a day; L/S ratio at 2/1; phosphatidylglycerol should be present; the lungs are now matured for normal function outside the uterus; end of the saccular period of lung development*
Weeks 38–42	Term birth; length 48–52 cm; weight 2.5–4 kg; heart rate 130–140 beats/min; respirations 30–50 breaths/min; blood pressure 75/40 mmHg; blood volume 80–100 mL/kg; stroke volume 4–5 mL/kg; VT 6–10 mL/kg; 50 million alveoli present; lung surface area 2.8 M²; Pores of Kohn are present

FETAL BREATHING, RESPIRATION, AND CIRCULATION

In utero, the lung of the fetus is filled with fluid. He or she does, however, make breathing motions that may move some fluid in and out of the lungs. This motion is associated with fetal well-being, helps with lung development, and is caused by diaphragm contraction. Respiration occurs in utero via the placenta with oxygen transferring from the maternal circulation to the fetal circulation and carbon dioxide going in the opposite direction. Fetal circulation is diagrammed and described in *Respiratory Care*. There are six major differences between fetal and adult circulation.

The fetus has the following:

1. A placental/umbilical circulation
2. An increased PO_2 in its venous system
3. A ductus venosus
4. A patent foramen ovale
5. A ductus arteriosus
6. Right-sided pressures (right atrium, right ventricle, pulmonary artery) are higher than left-sided pressures (left atrium, left ventricle, aorta)

THE GREAT TRANSITION—PART 1

When the fetus is born, his or her lungs are expected to make an immediate transition from a fluid-filled chamber to an air-breathing organ. This change in function is unparalleled by any other organ system. The fluid in the lungs is either drained (suctioned, squeezed) from the lungs, or it is absorbed from the lungs and removed via the lymphatics or the pulmonary circulation. The newborn must create a large negative pressure for his or her first breaths. These pressures may range from –20 to –80 cmH$_2$O. The reason for this large negative pressure is threefold. The fetus has to overcome the viscosity of the fluid in the lungs, overcome surface tension, and overcome tissue-resistant forces. As the lungs inflate, the amount of negative pressure required to breathe drops dramatically in a few breaths. This is made possible because, as alveoli inflate, surfactant is secreted from the type II cells and coats the alveolar surfaces. This decreases surface tension and stabilizes the alveoli. For a short period of time, as the newborn continues to breathe, he or she will have smaller exhaled volumes than inhaled volumes as he or she develops his or her functional residual capacity (FRC). Within 30 minutes, 95% of the newborn's FRC will be formed.

THE GREAT TRANSITION—PART 2

As described earlier, fetal circulation is different from adult circulation. At birth, as with the respiratory system, the circulatory system is also expected to make a dramatic transition in a very short period of time. There are several factors that are responsible for this transition. The first is lung expansion. Lung expansion allows air to fill the lung, increasing both the PAO_2 and the PaO_2. The lung expansion also results in a mechanical dilation of the pulmonary blood vessels.

The second factor is the clamping of the umbilical blood vessels. The placental circulation is a low resistance system. When the umbilical cord is clamped and cut, all aortic blood flow is forced through the systemic circulation of the newborn. The result is an increase in systemic or left-sided pressure.

The third factor involves ways of reducing right-sided pressure. The increased PaO_2 stimulates the release of several "chemicals" into the blood stream from the tissues. Prostaglandins E (PGE) and I, bradykinin, and nitric oxide (NO), along with the mechanical dilation and the increased PaO_2, dilate the pulmonary vessels and decrease pulmonary resistance. This high-resistance system with little blood flow in utero now becomes a low-resistance system with a lot of blood flow with a much lower pressure.

Because the left-sided pressure has increased some and right-sided pressure has decreased a lot, the foramen ovale will close. Remember that the foramen ovale is not just a hole but a door. As pressure increases on the left, compared with the right, the door swings shut. Functional closure will occur within a few minutes after birth. In moments of distress (hypoxemia), it is possible that the pressures will change and the foramen ovale will reopen. It may be months before the foramen anatomically seals. In some individuals, it never seals and can be opened as adults.

The last major factor in the transition of fetal to adult circulation is the closure of the ductus arteriosus. The increased PaO_2 and the release of PGF help constrict the ductus arteriosus. Functional closure will occur in a few hours and anatomic closure in a few days. During the time when it is open, blood will flow through it in the opposite direction of which it did in utero. This is because left-sided pressure is now higher than right-sided pressure.

The ductus venosus will also close in a few days. Both the ductus arteriosus and the ductus venosus will become permanent ligaments within the body.

NEWBORN ASSESSMENT

At the time of birth, the newborn must be assessed and some basic needs met. It has been suggested that, at the time of delivery, the 5 "Hs" must be resolved: hypoxemia, hypercarbia, hypotension, hypoglycemia, and hypothermia. One of the methods used in this process is the Apgar scoring system. The Apgar score, as described in *Respiratory Care*, is a five-area scoring system with each area scored from 0 to 2. A total of 0 to 10 points is possible. The Apgar system helps the physician to: identify depressed infants, assess severity of depression, initiate resuscitation appropriate to the level of depression, and allow immediate evaluation of the resuscitation efforts. For those who infrequently use the Apgar scoring system and forget the five areas of evaluation, the following acrostic may be helpful.

A	appearance	(color)
P	pulse	(heart rate)
G	grimace	(reflex irritability)
A	activity	(muscle tone)
R	respirations	(respiratory effort)

TEMPERATURE REGULATION IN THE NEWBORN

Although each of the 5 "Hs" could be addressed individually, I would like to spend just a little time discussing temperature regulation of the newborn or, in other words, preventing hypothermia. Heat loss can occur by the following four methods.

Radiant heat loss: The loss of body heat via electromagnetic waves to cooler objects that are not in direct contact with the body (a cold wall).

Convective heat loss: The loss of body heat owing to cooler air circulating over the body surface (cool gas flow into a hood).

Conductive heat loss: The loss of body heat owing to direct contact with cooler objects (cold hands on bare skin).

Evaporative heat loss: The loss of body heat as water evaporates and is converted into a vapor (not drying or covering a wet newborn baby).

Each of these methods of heat loss can present dangers to a newborn. What are some of the factors that affect the neonate's ability to maintain a constant body temperature?

1. Infants have an increased skin permeability (increased evaporation).
2. Infants have an increased percentage of body water (increased evaporation).
3. Infants have an increased surface area:body volume ratio. (The relatively large surface area will allow cooling to occur quickly, especially since there is such a small volume of heat reserve.)
4. Infants lack fat (fat is an insulator).
5. Infants do have brown fat. (Metabolism of brown fat is an exothermic reaction, that is, it produces

heat. Breakdown of brown fat is an important method of heat production in newborns. This process of producing heat is known as "nonshivering thermogenesis.")

6. Infants have the ability to shiver. (Shivering, or muscle twitching, will produce heat, but it also consumes much oxygen. The increase in metabolism is worse than the benefit of heat production for a newborn.)

7. Infants can regulate blood flow to their skin. (The automatic regulation of blood flow to the skin will conserve heat when needed or release heat if required.)

8. Infants do have the ability to sweat. (Sweat glands are functional in term newborns and will help in evaporative heat loss when required. Sweating is severely limited in premature infants.)

Routinely, overheating is not a major concern for newborns, although, it has been listed as a possible risk factor in the development of sudden infant death syndrome (SIDS). In general, infant cooling is a much greater concern. Hypothermia in infants has been shown to increase metabolism leading to hypoglycemia and hypoxemia/hypoxia; increase work of breathing; cause acidemia; and cause irregular respirations/apnea, resulting in increased mortality.

The following is a list of ways to help prevent heat loss in newborns.

1. Keep infants away from drafts.
2. Keep infants dry.
3. keep infants clothed or covered.
4. Place infants in an isolette (incubator).
5. Warm and humidify all gases delivered to infants.
6. Use a radiant heater when indicated.
7. Maintain a neutral thermal environment. This is the range of environmental temperatures in which a baby with a normal body temperature can maintain that temperature with a minimal metabolic rate. This temperature is different for babies of different sizes and ages. It also varies according to the amount of clothes the infant is wearing or the amount of coverings that are present.

HEMOGLOBIN AND THE OXYHEMOGLOBIN DISSOCIATION CURVE

There are more than 100 forms of hemoglobin (Hb). Normal adults have what is known as adult Hb (HbA). The fetus has fetal Hb (HbF) for most of its intrauterine life. Although the fetus has several types of Hb in embryonic and early fetal life, HbF makes up 95% of a fetus' Hb by week 10. The concentration is main-

tained at this level until week 30 at which time the fetus starts to manufacture HbA. By term birth, HbF has a concentration of 70% to 80% and HbA 20% to 30%. By 4 to 6 months after birth, HbA constitutes 95% of the Hb present. HbF shifts the oxyhemoglobin dissociation curve to the left. This means, when comparing the curves, that for a given PO_2, HbF will have a higher oxyHb saturation compared with HbA. Another way of putting it is to say that for any for a given oxyHb saturation, the fetal/newborn PO_2 will be lower compared with adult PO_2. The following chart illustrates this.

Approximate Comparisons for Normal Curves

OxyHb Saturation (%)	Adult PO_2 (mmHg)	Fetal/Newborn PO_2 (mmHg)
95	80	60
90	62	47
85	53	41
80	48	36
75	41	33
70	37	30
65	34	27
60	32	24
55	29	22
50	27	20

A PaO_2 of 60 mmHg in a newborn will result in an O_2Sat of 95%, whereas it takes a PaO_2 of 80 mmHg in the adult to achieve an O_2Sat of 95%. A PaO_2 of 33 mmHg in a newborn will result in an O_2Sat of 75%, whereas it takes a PaO_2 of 41 mmHg in the adult to achieve an O_2Sat of 75%. This is because the fetal oxyHb curve is shifted to the left.

The highest PO_2 that the fetal cells are exposed to is less than 30 mmHg. The systemic venous PO_2 values of the fetus are in the low teens. This is in contrast to the adult who normally has a PaO_2 in the range of 80 to 100 mmHg and a PvO_2 in the range of 40 mmHg. The following question could be raised: How does the fetus not only survive but grow and develop when exposed to such a low PO_2? There are several answers to this question.

First, the fetus has an increased Hb level. The fetus may have Hb levels of 19 g% and higher. This increased level will result in increased oxygen content.

Example

An adult with an oxyHb Sat of 98%, Hb of 13 g%, and a PaO_2 of 90 mmHg will have an oxygen content of 17.34 mL/100 mL of blood.

$$[(.98 \times 1.34 \times 13) + (.003 \times 90) = 17.34]$$

A fetus with an oxyHb Sat of 70%, a Hb of 19 g%, and a PO_2 of 30 mmHg will have an oxygen content of 17.91 mL/100 mL of blood.

$$[(.70 \times 1.34 \times 19) + (.003 \times 30)] = 17.91]$$

If the adult in the above example is the mother and the fetus her baby, it can be seen that the fetus actually has a higher oxygen content than his or her mother.

Second, the fetus can thrive in utero because HbF has an increased affinity for oxygen. That is, the oxyHb curve is shifted to the left. In the above example, a PO_2 of 30 resulted in a 70% oxyHb Sat for the fetus. If the adult would have had a PaO_2 of 30, their %Sat would have been 55%. The left shift again results in an increased oxygen content.

A third advantage for the fetus is that he or she is working on the steep portion of the oxyHb curve. In the adult, when the PO_2 drops from 80 to 40 mmHg, the %Sat decreases from 95% to 75%. This is a 20% oxygen content unloading from the Hb. In the fetus, when the PO_2 drops from 30 to 20 mmHg, the %Sat drops from 70% to 50%. This is also a 20% oxygen content unloading from the Hb, but HbF unloaded the same 20% with only a 10 mmHg change in the PO_2 instead of a 40 mmHg change required by HbA.

All this is showing is that much more oxygen is available to fetal tissue for a very small change in PO_2 compared with HbA.

The fourth advantage for the fetus is that the pH swing between arterial and venous blood is greater than that of normal adults. This change in pH promotes loading of oxygen at the placenta where the pH is higher. It also increases unloading at the fetal tissue where pH is lower (Bohr effect). This same effect is present in adults, but with a wider swing in pH, the effects are more exaggerated in the fetus and more oxygen is made available for consumption.

RESPIRATORY DISTRESS SYNDROME OF THE NEWBORN

Respiratory distress syndrome (RDS) of the newborn is discussed in *Respiratory Care*. I would like to add a few comments to the information listed there. There are four basic reasons for hypoxemia: shunt, $\dot{V}/\dot{Q}$ mismatch, diffusion defects, and hypoventilation. A newborn suffering from RDS can have all four of these problems. It is no wonder that infants afflicted with RDS do so poorly. Figure 25-1 illustrates each of the reasons for hypoxemia, and some of the factors involved.

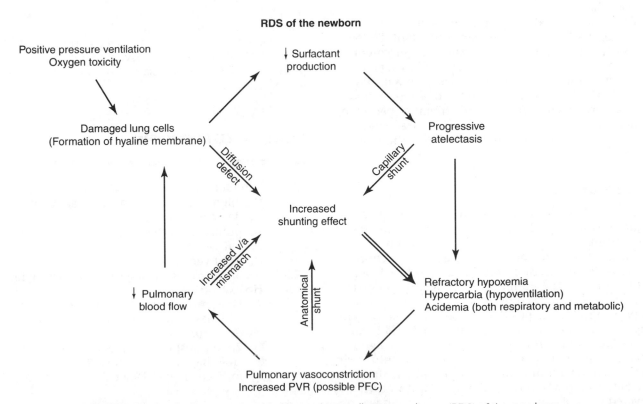

FIGURE 25-1. Cyclic events involved in respiratory distress syndrome (RDS) of the newborn.

CASE STUDIES

Case Study 1

P. B. is a 23-year-old pregnant woman with insulin-dependent diabetes mellitus and a positive smoking history. On 7/19 she presented to the hospital with evidence of pre-eclampsia and was treated with Betamethasone. She also developed some intermittent contractions, which were treated with Nifedipine. One week later, a repeat 24-hour urine test showed increasing proteinuria, and the decision was made to induce labor. Labor was not progressing, and external fetal monitoring revealed a flat tracing so a Cesarean delivery was performed.

B. B. was a 31-week premature female infant, weighing 1530 g. She was crying spontaneously but required a brief period of blow-by oxygen. She was a little floppy in the delivery room but had no significant RDS. An umbilical blood gas test revealed a pH of 7.26, $PaCO_2$ of 56 mmHg, PaO_2 of 13 mmHg, O_2Sat of 11%, and an HCO_3 of 25 mM/L. Apgar scores assigned at 1 and 5 minutes were 7 and 8, respectively. The infant was taken to NICU and placed on nasal continuous positive airway pressure (CPAP) of +5 cmH_2O following significant desaturations and prolonged apnea spells. Chest radiographs revealed findings consistent with a diagnosis of hyaline membrane disease (HMD). B. B. was also started on Ampicillin and Gentamicin for possible sepsis. An umbilical catheter was placed for blood sampling, and B. B. was made NPO (nothing by mouth) and placed on intravenous fluids.

The next day B. B. was intubated with a 3.0 endotracheal tube (ETT) to administer surfactant. Following surfactant therapy, B. B.'s oxygen requirement was reduced from 40% to 23%. The following day, B. B. was extubated and placed back on nasal CPAP of +5 cmH_2O. She remained on CPAP of +5 for 2 more days and received caffeine for treatment of periods of apnea. When CPAP was removed, B. B. was able to maintain oxygenation and ventilation without assistance.

Case Study 2

G. S. is a 620-g, 24-week preterm infant born to a 22-year-old woman with a positive history of smoking and asthma. The mother presented to the hospital on 5/8 with back pain. Following a diagnosis of chorioamnionitis, the decision was made to induce labor.

G. S. presented with moderate RDS and cyanosis but had spontaneous movements. The infant's color improved following positive pressure ventilation with bag and mask. Apgar scores assigned at 1 and 5 minutes were 6 and 7, respectively. However, owing to persistent poor ventilatory effort, G. S. was intubated in the delivery room with a 2.5 ETT and transferred to the NICU. G. S. was admitted to a radiant warmer and covered with plastic wrap. A chest radiograph was ob-tained, and it was consistent with HMD. G. S. was placed on a ventilator with a rate of 40/min, peak inspiratory pressure (PIP) of 20 cmH_2O, positive end-expiratory pressure (PEEP) of +5 cmH_2O, and 60% oxygen. Survanta was then delivered via the ETT. Response to the surfactant was favorable and the FIO_2 was decreased from 60% to 35%. Arterial blood gas (ABG) tests revealed a pH of 7.22, $PaCO_2$ of 55 mmHg, and a PaO_2 of 85 mmHg on 35% oxygen. G. S. received a second dose of Survanta 24 hours after the initial dose was given. Transfusions were also done because of the development of anemia secondary to phlebotomy and early jaundice of prematurity.

On May 11, G. S. was diagnosed with a nonclinically evident patent ductus arteriosus, and as a result, Indocin was started. An ultrasound study of the head revealed a small intracranial bleed.

Over the course of G. S.'s admission, fluid balance and calorie intake were of concern. G. S. became azotemic and hypernatremic within the first few days. G. S.'s weight gain was slow and remained a concern. G. S. was over 1 month old before he weighed 2 lb.

Within the first week, G. S.'s lung disease worsened. An ABG test on a rate of 60, PIP of 17 cmH_2O, PEEP of +4 cmH_2O, and 70% oxygen revealed a pH of 7.14, $PaCO_2$ of 59 mmHg, and a PaO_2 of 59 mmHg. Chest radiograph at this time showed diffuse densities in the right middle and lower lobes and the left lower lobe. In response to these findings, G. S. was started on Vancomycin and Gentamicin, albuterol, and chest physiotherapy.

Over the next several weeks, with the resolution of the patient's pneumonia and the patient's increased maturity, he was weaned from the ventilator. On 6/18, G. S. was extubated and placed on nasal CPAP of +5 cmH_2O and room air. Five days later he was placed on 0.025 L/min nasal cannula and discharged to home.

REVIEW QUESTIONS

25-1. Which of the following structures would have the highest PO_2 value in the fetal circulation?
   A. descending aorta
   B. pulmonary artery
   C. left ventricle
   D. right ventricle

25-2. All of the following are true concerning fetal Hb except:
   A. HbF shifts the oxyHb curve to the left
   B. HbF has a greater affinity for oxygen than does HbA
   C. 2,3-diphosphoglycerate binds better with HbF than it does with HbA
   D. for a given PO_2, HbF will have a higher %Sat than HbA

25-3. Endothelium relaxing factor (EDRF) has been identified as:
   A. guanylate cyclase
   B. cyclic guanosine 3,5'-monophosphate (cGMP)
   C. calcium
   D. nitric oxide

25-4. The best possible score when using the Apgar scoring system is:
   A. 1
   B. 2
   C. 5
   D. 10

25-5. Each of the following are assessed on the Apgar system except:
   A. pulse strength
   B. muscle tone
   C. respirations
   D. color

25-6. All of the following are correct except:
   A. phosphatidylglycerol presence in amniotic fluid predicts lung maturity 100% of the time
   B. absence of phosphatidylglycerol does not predict lung immaturity
   C. a 2:1 lecithin/sphingomyelin ratio will correctly predict lung maturity even in infants of diabetic mothers
   D. the L/S ratio cannot be performed with blood-contaminated amniotic fluid

25-7. Appropriate CPAP therapy will most likely have all of the following effects except:
   A. increased functional residual capacity
   B. redistribution of alveolar fluid into the interstitium
   C. decreased venous return
   D. decreased static lung compliance

25-8. Formation of the segmental bronchi marks the end of which period of lung development?
   A. embryonic
   B. pseudoglandular
   C. canalicular
   D. saccular

25-9. The entire bronchial tree (conducting airways) is formed by the end of which period of lung development?
   A. embryonic
   B. pseudoglandular
   C. canalicular
   D. saccular

25-10. The beginning of formation of the gas-exchange unit, the acinus, occurs during which weeks of lung development?
   A. 6 to 16
   B. 17 to 28
   C. 29 to 36
   D. 37 to 42

25-11. The alveolar period of lung development begins at 37 weeks and lasts until which of the following?
   A. birth
   B. 28 days after birth
   C. 2 years of age
   D. 8 years of age or older

25-12. Surfactant is synthesized, stored, and secreted by which type of lung cell?
   A. type I
   B. type II
   C. type III
   D. goblet cells

25-13. All of the following are correct concerning surface tension (ST) except:
   A. surfactant helps to decrease ST
   B. ST is greatest at end exhalation
   C. normally small alveoli are very stable
   D. limited amounts of surfactant will result in a decreased compliance

25-14. Each of the following accelerate fetal lung maturation except:
   A. corticosteroids
   B. thyroid hormones
   C. theophylline
   D. testosterone

25-15. Which of the following would be at higher risk for delayed lung maturation?
   A. a fetus with a diabetic mother
   B. fetus of black ethnic background
   C. fetus of female gender
   D. fetus exposed to placental insufficiency

25-16. In fetal circulation, which of the following allow shunting of blood directly from the pulmonary artery to the aorta?
   A. ductus venosus
   B. foramen ovale
   C. ductus arteriosus
   D. placenta

25-17. A full-term fetus would be born after how many weeks gestation?
   A. 32 to 34
   B. 35 to 37
   C. 38 to 42
   D. 43 to 45

25-18. Within minutes after birth, there is normal functional closure of which of the following?
   A. ductus arteriosus
   B. ductus venosus
   C. foramen ovale
   D. all of the above

25-19. When the umbilical cord is cut at birth, there should be present:
   A. 2 arteries, 1 vein
   B. 1 artery, 2 veins
   C. 1 artery, 1 vein
   D. 2 arteries, 2 veins

25-20. If measured, a newborn's first breaths would have a larger inhaled volume than exhaled volume. This is caused by which of the following?
   A. development of pulmonary interstitial emphysema
   B. formation of the functional residual capacity
   C. air leaks in the lungs
   D. the negative inspiratory force created

25-21. Which of the following are true concerning congenital diaphragmatic hernia?
   A. it usually occurs on the left side
   B. mortality is low (<20%) especially when extracorporeal membrane oxygenation (ECMO) is used
   C. surgery is rarely required
   D. bag-mask ventilation is preferred over endotracheal intubation

25-22. A newborn presents with RDS, breath sounds are diminished on the right and bowel sounds are heard on the left. The most likely diagnosis is:
   A. T-E fistula
   B. pulmonary interstitial emphysema
   C. RDS
   D. congenital diaphragmatic hernia

26

Respiratory Care for the Infant and Child

CASE STUDY

A 23-year-old woman, pregnant with her first child, was vacationing in Florida. While visiting Disney World, she started having uterine contractions. She was transported and admitted to a local hospital where labor could not be stopped, and a 26-week-gestation baby boy (O. M.) was born. His Apgar scores at 1 and 5 minutes were 2 and 3, respectively. O. M. was resuscitated, intubated, and placed on mechanical ventilation. Because of his prematurity, Survanta (surfactant) was given on two separate occasions. O. M. was diagnosed as having respiratory distress syndrome (RDS) of the newborn. He also presented with a patent ductus arteriosus (PDA), which was treated with Indocin, and hyperbilirubinemia, for which he received phototherapy. He also had a small intracranial bleed, which resolved, and he developed retinopathy of prematurity (ROP).

From the onset of mechanical ventilation, O. M. developed a left pneumothorax. Each time the chest tube was removed the lung would again collapse. After repeated attempts of inflating the lung using chest tubes, a left thoracotomy was performed to locate a bronchopleural fistula. This procedure resulted in a resection of the left upper lobe.

Since they were unable to wean O. M. from mechanical ventilation and oxygen, and with radiographic evidence, on day 39 O. M. was given the diagnosis of bronchopulmonary dysplasia (BPD). On day 50, the last chest tube was removed and the lung remained inflated. Chest radiograph revealed cystic areas, and the patient was diagnosed

with having pulmonary interstitial emphysema (PIE). Finally, after 2 months of mechanical ventilation and oxygen therapy, O. M. was weaned from the ventilator and placed on nasal cannula. Once the infant was stable and was able to be discharged, he and his mother returned to their home in the northeastern United States.

At 4 months of age, O. M. was admitted to the hospital with respiratory distress. He was treated with albuterol aerosol, aminophylline, and RespiGam. Premature infants with chronic pulmonary disease, like BPD, have a high incidence of respiratory syncytial virus (RSV) infections, which require hospitalization and extensive treatment. RespiGam is an RSV immunoglobulin administered intravenously (RSV-IGIV). The goal of administration of RespiGam is to prevent RSV infections or to decrease the severity of infection in those who do acquire an RSV infection. Infusions will be given once a month for 5 months during the RSV season. O. M. has received the first two of his five infusions and is tolerating them well.

REVIEW QUESTIONS

26-1. Each of the following is correct except:
A. an infant will preferentially breathe through its nose
B. the cricoid forms the narrowest point of the infant's upper airway
C. by age 6 years, children have an upper airway that resembles an adult's
D. the epiglottis is wider and more horizontally positioned in an infant than it is in an adult

26-2. Each of the following may indicate the need for suctioning except:
A. visible secretions in the endotracheal (ET) tube
B. presence of rhonchi
C. decreased pressures required to deliver a set V_T with mechanical ventilation
D. acute onset of dyspnea

26-3. The most common side effect on ET tube suctioning in infants and children is:
A. bradycardia
B. atelectasis
C. mucosal damage
D. infection

26-4. A guide for determining the appropriate V_T to deliver to a child during mechanical ventilation is:
A. 3 to 5 mL/kg
B. 5 to 10 mL/kg
C. 10 to 15 mL/kg
D. 15 to 20 mL/kg

26-5. During extubation, the ET tube should be removed:
  A. at end exhalation
  B. at end inspiration
  C. at mid inspiration
  D. at mid exhalation

26-6. Children with croup often have a neck radiograph depicting subglottic narrowing known as:
  A. the thumb sign
  B. the tunnel sign
  C. the steeple sign
  D. the pyramid sign

26-7. A child with an acute onset of sore throat, drooling, fever, and anxiety is most likely suffering from:
  A. croup
  B. epiglottitis
  C. asthma
  D. bronchiolitis

26-8. It appears that early treatment of bronchiolitis with ribavirin may result in each of the following except:
  A. decreased length of time mechanical ventilation is required
  B. decreased amount of supplemental oxygen required
  C. decreased length of stay in hospital
  D. decreased mortality rates

26-9. The probability of a child being born with cystic fibrosis, when only one parent is a carrier of the cystic fibrosis gene, is:
  A. 0%
  B. 25%
  C. 33%
  D. 50%

26-10. Which of the following groups have been listed at increased risk for submersion injuries?
  A. child <4 years of age supervised by one parent
  B. child <4 years of age supervised by two parents
  C. adolescent males between 15 and 19 years of age
  D. all of the above

26-11. Which of the following sites is most often involved with submersion injuries for pediatric patients?
  A. bath tubs
  B. swimming pools
  C. rivers
  D. ponds

26-12. The most important clinical complication of submersion injury is:
  A. increased fluid volume
  B. electrolyte imbalance
  C. hypoxemia
  D. pulmonary edema

26-13. Aspiration of water would result in each of the following except:
  A. inactivation of surfactant
  B. destruction of capillary endothelial cells
  C. increased compliance
  D. intrapulmonary shunting

26-14. Each of the following is correct except:
  A. children have a lower absolute blood volume than adults
  B. children are at greater risk for hypovolemia than adults
  C. initially with blood loss, children are unable to maintain a normal blood pressure
  D. with significant blood loss, children will rapidly decompensate with significant hypotension

26-15. Each of the following are true regarding smoke inhalation except:
  A. patients with smoke inhalation should be given 100% oxygen
  B. 100% oxygen should be given until COHb levels are <10%
  C. measuring COHb is the best method to evaluate oxygenation status
  D. it is appropriate to monitor SpO2 to evaluate oxygenation status with smoke inhalation

27

Bronchial Asthma

27-1. Write a definition of asthma in your own words. _____

_____

_____

_____

ASTHMA DRUGS

New asthma medications are slowly coming into the United States market. One of the most recent to be introduced is Serevent. Serevent (salmeterol xinafoate) is a highly selective beta$_2$-adrenergic aerosolized bronchodilator for oral inhalation. The metered-dose inhaler (MDI) delivers 21 µg from the activator with each activation. Serevent is a long-acting bronchodilator with a recommended dose of 2 puffs, twice a day (every 12 hours, morning and evening) and should *not* be taken more often. Serevent is to be used for maintenance treatment of asthma and should not be introduced for acutely deteriorating asthma or treatment of acute symptoms.

Another "drug" that can be used in the treatment of asthma is helium. Helium is a low-density gas (0.18 g/L) compared with air (1.29 g/L) or oxygen (1.43 g/L). Helium may be useful for treating increased airway resistance, which occurs during bronchoconstriction in asthma. According to Poiseuille's Law, airflow will increase and resistance will decrease as gas density decreases, if other factors remain constant. Using a mixture of helium and oxygen (heliox) should help asthma patients breathe more easily and ventilate better when having an acute attack. It can be delivered by a tight-fitting non-rebreathing mask or given to patients who require mechanical ventilation. It should be delivered by a blender system so that precise concentration of helium and oxygen can be given. Oxygen flowmeters used to deliver the helium mixture will not record accurate flow, since they are calibrated to deliver a higher density gas. Actual flow rates can be determined, but in general, flows will be higher than indicated.

CASE STUDIES

Case Study 1

M. R. is a 10-year-old girl who has mild asthma but is asymptomatic most of the time. Acute symptoms are routinely being treated with albuterol syrup, prescribed by her family physician. One afternoon, after playing outside in a dusty environment, she complained of increased shortness of breath and difficulty breathing. As usual, the albuterol syrup was given, but the breathing difficulties continued. Because her breathing did not improve, her parents brought M. R. to the hospital's emergency department.

On admission, M. R. was found to be a well-developed 10-year-old in moderate respiratory distress. Her peak flow (PF) was 90 L/min, respiratory rate 40, heart rate 140, and she had bilateral wheezing. A small volume nebulizer aerosol treatment was ordered with 0.5 mL (2.5 mg) of albuterol in 3 mL of saline. Thirty minutes after the treatment, M. R. said she was feeling much better. Her PF had improved to 200 L/min, heart rate was 120, respiratory rate was 25, and all but a few distant wheezes had disappeared. Following observation for one hour, M. R. was discharged. Before discharge, M. R. and her parents were instructed in the use of an albuterol MDI. They were also referred for follow-up evaluation by a pulmonary specialist.

M. R. had a dramatic improvement and no further follow-up was needed.

Case Study 2

D. B. is a 30-year-old man with a known history of asthma since age 2 years. He has been symptom free until 2 months ago when hospitalized and treated successfully without intubation. He has allergies to eggs, sulfa drugs, animal dander, molds, ragweed, dust, pollen, and so forth. Current medications include Proventil Inhaler and Theo-Dur 300 mg twice a day. D. B. was visiting the area and staying in a hotel. It is unknown if he was exposed to an allergin. He said his symptoms started at noon after giving a martial arts demonstration. His symptoms had progressively worsened even with the use of his inhaler, and he is now seeking medical help in the hospital emergency department.

D. B. presented in the emergency department

around 8 PM with severe respiratory distress. Respiratory rate of 48, pulse of 134, blood pressure of 158/84, and SpO_2 of 93% on 4 L/min nasal cannula. There were audible wheezes on inspiration and expiration. Sternal retractions were present. Radiograph showed hyperaeration. The patient denied coughing and was unable to perform a peak flow but was fully alert and cooperative. Over the next 30 minutes, the patient was given the following medications. Three consecutive aerosol treatments via small-volume nebulizer (SVN) with 2.5 mg of albuterol in 3.5 mL of solution, 60 mg of prednisone, 2 g of magnesium sulfate in 100 mL of normal saline solution intravenously, and 80 mg Solu-Medrol intravenously. At this point, the patient was having minimal relief and, with movement, experienced desaturations. He was placed on a nonrebreathing mask and an arterial blood gas (ABG) test was performed. pH = 7.32, $PaCO_2$ = 50 mmHg, HCO_3 = 26 mM/L, PaO_2 = 273 mmHg, O_2Sat = 100%. Following the ABG, the patient was started on heliox and a fourth aerosol treatment was given with heliox. The patient remained stable and said that his breathing was easier. The patient continued to improve over the next 2 hours and was then transferred to a hospital room. At the time of transfer, the heliox was discontinued. His respiratory rate was 18, pulse was 105, BP was 130/72, and SpO_2 was 98%. The patient plan was to continue the present medications and taper them as he showed continued improvement. Oxygen was to be titrated to keep SpO_2 at >93%. That evening, his PF was 190 L/min and increased to 260 L/min following an aerosol treatment. D. B. continued to improve and was discharged 2 days later. On discharge, his PF was >360 L/min.

D. B. had a severe asthma attack. His arterial blood gas tests revealed a respiratory acidemia and tracheal intubation was considered. Whether it was the heliox or the other medications kicking in that resulted in the improvement is unknown, but because the patient started to improve almost immediately after instituting heliox, tracheal intubation was adverted.

REVIEW QUESTIONS

27-2. Each of the following characterize asthma except:
   A. reversible airway obstruction
   B. airway inflammation
   C. decreased airway resistance
   D. increased airway responsiveness to stimuli
27-3. Each of the following are present in severe asthma except:
   A. overdistended lungs
   B. decreased eosinophiles
   C. epithelial cells present in airway mucus
   D. mucus plugging

27-4. The predominant airway response to an antigen soon after aerosol challenge is which of the following?
   A. bronchospasm
   B. mucus production
   C. swelling (edema)
   D. cellular inflammation
27-5. An airway challenge test uses which of the following for documentation?
   A. peak flow
   B. forced vital capacity (FVC)
   C. forced expiratory volume in 1 second (FEV_1)
   D. forced expiratory flow FEF_{25-75}
27-6. Airway hyper-responsiveness to methacholine is expressed as the concentration of agent required to produce what percent drop in FEV_1?
   A. 10%
   B. 20%
   C. 30%
   D. 40%
27-7. Asthma management may include all of the following except:
   A. immunotherapy
   B. inhaled corticosteroids
   C. oral cromolyn
   D. allergen avoidance
27-8. Each of the following characterize severe asthma except:
   A. decreased expiratory flow rates
   B. ventilation-perfusion inequality
   C. hypoxemia
   D. hypocapnia
27-9. Which of the following is the most reliable for documentation of severity of airflow obstruction?
   A. caregivers' subjective findings
   B. physical examination
   C. pulmonary function studies
   D. patient's subjective feelings
27-10. An improvement of what percent in FEV_1 following bronchodilator is considered significant and supports the diagnosis of asthma?
   A. 10%
   B. 15%
   C. 20%
   D. 25%
27-11. Which of the following pulmonary function parameters is considered to be most effort dependent?
   A. peak flow
   B. FEV_1
   C. FEF_{25-75}
   D. FEV_1/FVC
27-12. Initially, a patient suffering from an intermediate asthma attack will demonstrate which acid-base disorder?
   A. respiratory acidemia
   B. respiratory alkalemia
   C. metabolic acidemia
   D. metabolic alkalemia

27-13. The first choice of therapy for acute asthma is most often recommended as which of the following?
   A. subcutaneous injection of bronchodilators
   B. intravenous bronchodilator therapy
   C. continuous aerosol administration of bronchodilators
   D. episodic aerosol administration of bronchodilators

27-14. The major benefit of hospitalization for asthma is:
   A. availability of continuous aerosol administration
   B. the use of injectable bronchodilators
   C. the use of systemic steroids
   D. the availability of close observation and rapid intervention if needed

27-15. A patient with acute severe asthma should be considered for endotracheal intubation once their $PaCO_2$ is greater than what value?
   A. 30 mmHg
   B. 40 mmHg
   C. 50 mmHg
   D. 60 mmHg

27-16. All of the following contribute significantly to asthma mortality except:
   A. underestimating asthma severity
   B. undertreatment with corticosteroids
   C. overtreatment with aminophylline
   D. delay in seeking medical care

28

Chronic Obstructive Pulmonary Disease

CASE STUDY

J. C. is a 67-year-old man with end-stage severe chronic obstructive pulmonary disease (COPD), chronic bronchitis, bullous emphysema, and cor pulmonale. He has a 100 pack/year smoking history but stopped smoking 5 years ago. He has had several hospital admissions in the past years. Twenty years ago, he had a right lung adenocarcinoma resected; 12 years ago, he was classified as totally disabled by his pulmonary disease; and 5 years ago, he was intubated and mechanically ventilated owing to ventilatory failure. He was weaned from the ventilator after a long period of time. Following this hospitalization, he became oxygen dependent and is now on 2 L/min constantly.

His present hospitalization is caused by an exacerbation of his COPD with increased shortness of breath, decreased physical activity, and depression. His condition had progressed to the point where he was basically living out of his recliner. He was unable to care for himself (eg, bathing) or walk any distance without extreme dyspnea. The goal of the admission was to treat the acute exacerbation, maximize his pulmonary toilet, and increase his endurance for activities of daily living.

On admission, J. C. was somewhat lethargic but a good historian. It was difficult for him to communicate because of his dyspnea. He had a chronic cough with little expectoration. His arterial blood gas (ABG) test revealed a respiratory acidemia with a pH of 7.27 and a $PaCO_2$ of 75 mmHg. His drugs included Zantec, Synthroid,

Theo-Dur, Bumex, Prednisone, Albuterol, Atrovent, oxygen, and antibiotics.

After a week of aggressive respiratory, physical, and emotional therapy, J. C. showed signs of improvement. He was able to bathe himself and walk 140 feet with oxygen. His forced expiratory volume in 1 second (FEV_1) was 0.5 L (16% of predicted, same as on admission). His ABG on 2 L/min nasal cannula was pH = 7.34, $PaCO_2$ = 59 mmHg, PaO_2 = 65 mmHg. J. C. was discharged from the hospital, the goals being met. There is concern, however, that with his end-stage disease, there is little that can be done medically for this gentleman in the future.

REVIEW QUESTIONS

28-1. The diagnosis of COPD is typically made by each of the following methods except:
   A. radiographic appearance
   B. lung tissue sample
   C. patient history
   D. pulmonary function testing

28-2. The most important pathologic abnormality in the major airways of patients with COPD is:
   A. smooth muscle hypertrophy
   B. bronchial wall thickness
   C. bronchial wall inflammation
   D. mucus gland hyperplasia and hypersecretion

28-3. Emphysematous lungs have expiratory airflow obstruction due to which of the following:
   A. increased chest wall compliance
   B. decreased lung compliance
   C. increased lung elasticity
   D. decreased tethering

28-4. Antiprotease deficiency is estimated to account for what percent of the emphysema cases in the United States?
   A. 1%
   B. 5%
   C. 8%
   D. 15%

28-5. All of the following are true except:
   A. emphysema in smokers is centrilobular
   B. emphysema in antiprotease deficiency is panacinar (panlobular)
   C. differentiation of the two types of emphysema is clinically important
   D. degree of airflow obstruction is a function of severity of emphysema, not type

28-6. The predominant risk factor for the development of COPD in the industrialized world is:
   A. smoking
   B. dust exposure
   C. fumes and gas
   D. prior pulmonary disease

28-7. Factors that influence survival of COPD patients are listed below. Which of the following is not considered one of the most important?
   A. FEV$_1$
   B. patient's age
   C. response to bronchodilator
   D. whether or not the patient continues to smoke

28-8. Dyspnea is defined as:
   A. the caregivers' objective evaluation of the patient
   B. the caregivers' subjective evaluation of the patient
   C. the patient's subjective evaluation of his breathing
   D. a respiratory rate of greater than 30 breaths per minute

28-9. Which of the following physical findings is not routinely present in advanced COPD?
   A. barrel chest
   B. digital clubbing
   C. use of accessory respiratory muscles
   D. prolonged exhalation

28-10. By definition, COPD patients have:
   A. a decreased forced vital capacity
   B. a decreased FEV$_1$
   C. an increased functional residual capacity
   D. an increased total lung capacity

28-11. Each of the following show evidence of lung hyperinflation except:
   A. hyperlucent lung fields
   B. flattened diaphragms
   C. prominent interstitial markings
   D. increased retrosternal airspace

28-12. Approximately what percent of lung cancers are attributable to cigarette smoking?
   A. <50%
   B. 75%
   C. 90%
   D. 99.9%

28-13. Which of the following is classified as an anti-inflammatory drug?
   A. cromolyn
   B. theophylline
   C. atrovent
   D. albuterol

28-14. Use of which of the following drugs for treatment of pulmonary has demonstrated improved survival in patients with COPD?
   A. beta agonists
   B. oxygen
   C. prostaglandins
   D. all of the above

28-15. The primary determinant of ventilatory failure in patients with COPD is:
   A. viral infections
   B. increased sputum production
   C. bacterial infections
   D. respiratory muscle fatigue

28-16. Which of the following are proven treatment for COPD patients with nocturnal hypoxemia?
   A. oxygen
   B. acetazolamide
   C. theophylline
   D. all of the above

_____

_____

_____

Using a ventilation monitor, record the following:

Breathing frequency, tidal volume, and vital capacity

_____

_____

_____

CASE STUDY

J. E. is a 27-year-old woman who is 65 inches tall and weighs 506 lb. She has a history of asthma with at least one previous admission for respiratory difficulty, which resolved quickly. She has a restrictive lung disorder with a forced vital capacity (FVC) of 65% of her predicted value and an FEV_1/FVC ratio of 0.95. She also has a history of sleep apnea with oxygen desaturation. A room air sleep study revealed a mean O_2Sat of 87% and a low of 76% during sleep. A repeat study on 1 L/min nasal cannula resulted in a mean O_2Sat of 92% and a low of 81%. Home oxygen was ordered for sleep.

Recent medical history is unremarkable and uneventful except that 2 weeks before admission, J. E. had a fever and cold symptoms and was treated by her family physician. She had no recent immunizations. J. E. was admitted to the emergency department on 3/12/96 at 12:30 PM. She complained of increasing muscle weakness and numbness of her hands and feet, which had started 3 days earlier. She stated that "it feels like it is coming up my body and now even the muscles I use to breathe don't seem to be working." Her respiratory assessment included a VC of 2.4 L (pred 4.2 L), frequency of 24 breaths/min, PImax of −58 cmH_2O, and her lungs were clear. A room air arterial blood gas (ABG) study revealed a normal acid-base status with mild hypoxemia. pH = 7.44, $PaCO_2$ = 36 mmHg, and PaO_2 = 66 mmHg. She was negative for diplopia (double vision), dysphagia (difficulty in swallowing), dysphasia (impairment of speech), and ptosis (drooping eyelids). She was, however, feeling very depressed and seemed emotionally unstable.

Following her emergency department assessment, it was decided to admit J. E. to the intensive care unit for close observation. Over the next 4 hours, she complained of increased feelings of fatigue. A re-assessment of her respiratory parameters revealed the fol-

29

Neuromuscular Disease

STUDENT EXERCISES

29-1. Inspiratory muscle strength is important for what reasons? _____

_____

_____

_____

29-2. Expiratory muscle strength is important for what reasons? _____

_____

_____

_____

Laboratory Exercises

29-3. Using a manometer and appropriate adapters, measure the following:

PImax at residual volume, functional residual capacity (FRC), and near total lung capacity (TLC). Does lung volume level affect the ability to generate pressure?

_____

_____

_____

lowing: VC decreased to 1.5 L (from 2.4 L), PImax decreased to −30 cmH$_2$O (from −58 cmH$_2$O), and respiratory rate increased to 36 breaths/min (from 24). Based on this data and the patients worsening clinical appearance, an elective intubation was performed.

The patient was initially set up on assist/control, volume-cycled mechanical ventilation with a frequency of 10/min, Vt of 750 mL, FiO$_2$ of 60%, and +3 cmH$_2$O of positive end-expiratory pressure (PEEP). An ABG analysis 20 minutes after stabilization showed a respiratory acidemia with a pH of 7.27, a PaCO$_2$ of 58 mmHg, and a PaO$_2$ of 80 mmHg. Respiratory frequency was increased to 16 breaths/min and her ABG normalized. Over the next several days, her ventilator settings were maintained as follows: frequency = 16 breaths/min, Vt = 750 to 800 mL, FiO$_2$ = 50% to 65%, and PEEP = +7 cmH$_2$O. The peak inspiratory pressure (PIP) during her entire course of ventilation ranged from 28 to 35 cmH$_2$O and her lung-thorax compliance ranged from 30 to 40 mL/cmH$_2$O. Early in the course of her stay, she would become very restless with head and neck movement but rarely cycled the ventilator. Failure to calm the patient resulted in administration of some sedation. For the next 2 months, she would fluctuate between following and not following commands but rarely opened her eyes. When following commands, she would communicate by shaking her head slightly or moving her eyebrows in response to questions.

On the day following admission (3/13/96), an electromyogram (nerve conduction study) was done. The test was positive for a demyelinating polyneuropathy, and the patient was assigned a diagnosis of Guillain-Barré syndrome (GBS). A second test 2 days (3/15/96) later demonstrated the same results. Because of the patient's size and suspected need for long-term ventilation, indirect calorimetry was performed 3 days after admission (3/15/96). Her VO$_2$ was 462 mL/min and her resting energy expenditure was 3211 kcal/day. Repeat studies on 3/22/96 and 3/29/96 revealed slightly higher, but approximately the same, results. Because of her hypermetabolic state, she was observed very closely nutritionally throughout her stay. Respiratory parameters were performed daily, but little change was seen from day to day. After 5 days of mechanical ventilation, she had a VC of 246 mL and a PImax of −5 cmH$_2$O. Owing to her lack of improvement and probable need for long-term ventilation, the decision was made to perform a tracheotomy.

During this same time period, J. E.'s blood pressure was unstable with the pressure fluctuating up and down. She also developed pupillary dysfunction. A CAT scan of her head was done to check for a cerebral infarct, but it was negative. The blood pressure and pupillary instability were most likely caused by dysfunction of the autonomic nervous system, which is common in GBS.

Seven days following admission (3/19/96), J. E. developed a right lower lobe pneumonia. Because of the patient's size, it was difficult to provide adequate postural drainage therapy. She was treated with appropriate antibiotic therapy, and 3 days later (3/22/96) a therapeutic bronchoscopy was performed. The pneumonic process seemed to peak on 3/23/96 with a patient temperature of 107°F. The patient's ventilator settings on this day were frequency of 26, Vt of 800, FiO$_2$ of 100%, and PEEP of +12 cmH$_2$O. Over the next 4 days, the patient improved, and by 3/27/96 the FiO$_2$ was decreased to 40%. By 4/8/96 the patient was back on a frequency of 16 breaths/min, Vt of 800 mL, FiO$_2$ of 40%, and PEEP of +10 cmH$_2$O.

One of the treatments for GBS is plasma exchange (hemapheresis). The goal of hemapheresis is to remove autoimmune factors from the blood to help alleviate the patient's signs and symptoms. In the process, blood products (cells) are separated from the plasma. The plasma, containing the autoimmune factors, is removed and disposed. The blood products are mixed with replacement plasma and returned to the patient. J. E. received three plasma exchange treatments early in the course of the disease, but it did not appear to result in any immediate improvement in her clinical condition. There was even concern that the plasma exchanges were having a negative impact on her acute clinical course and they were discontinued.

Following 3 months of very slow progress, J. E. was alert and responding appropriately by moving her head in response to questions. In early June, some spontaneous ventilation was noted. J. E., having been on A/C ventilation, was now (6/5/96) placed on SIMV of 10, PS of +14, with 30-minute trach collar trials (40% oxygen) three times daily as tolerated. By 6/18/96, J. E. was on SIMV only at night with trach collar trials during the day. On 6/20/96, the ventilator was discontinued and J. E. was placed on continuous trach collar at 40% oxygen. The use of a Passey-Muir valve was instituted, with the trach tube cuff deflated, to allow for speech. An ABG analysis showed normal acid-base balance and oxygenation. Volume-oriented intermittent positive pressure breathing (IPPB) treatments were given every 4 hours with 1.2 to 1.6 L. On 7/16/96, J. E. was transferred to a long-term care facility. ABGs were normal and chest radiograph showed decreased lung volumes with some basilar atelectasis. At date of discharge, J. E. was being placed out of bed into a wheel chair. She still weighed 492 lb. She was able to talk, but it was often difficult to understand her. She was unable to move her extremities except her head and neck. It is unknown how much functional movement will return and only time will tell.

REVIEW QUESTIONS

29-4. The primary source of the inspiratory signal to the respiratory muscles is the:
   A. upper pons
   B. lower pons
   C. medulla
   D. cortex

29-5. The central chemoreceptors are located where?
   A. in the pons
   B. near the surface of the medulla
   C. in the ventricles of the brain
   D. in the capillary walls of the vessels of the cortex

29-6. The central chemoreceptors are responsive to:
   A. $PaCO_2$
   B. arterial pH
   C. the $[H^+]$ of the extracellular fluid of the medulla
   D. cerebrospinal fluid PCO_2

29-7. Peripheral chemoreceptors respond to:
   A. arterial pH
   B. PaO_2
   C. $PaCO_2$
   D. all of the above

29-8. Increased $PaCO_2$ results in:
   A. increased intracranial pressure (ICP)
   B. decreased cerebral blood flow
   C. cerebral vasoconstriction
   D. all of the above

29-9. Severe heart failure commonly results in what abnormal breathing pattern?
   A. hypoventilation
   B. apneustic breathing
   C. Cheyne-Stokes breathing
   D. ataxic breathing

29-10. A breathing pattern characterized by prolonged cessation of breathing in the inspiratory position is:
   A. central sleep apnea
   B. apneustic breathing
   C. Cheyne-Stokes breathing
   D. ataxic breathing

29-11. Phrenic nerve pacemakers would be indicated in:
   A. cluster breathing
   B. central sleep apnea
   C. ataxic breathing
   D. central neurogenic hyperventilation

29-12. Each of the following are true concerning quadriplegia with spared diaphragmatic function except:
   A. the diaphragm must increase its level of work
   B. there is an increased risk of respiratory complications
   C. the ability to cough is maintained
   D. inspiratory capacity may be good

29-13. *Campylobacter jejuni* has been implicated in which of the following diseases?
   A. amyotrophic lateral sclerosis
   B. GBS
   C. polio
   D. myasthenia gravis (MG)

29-14. Which of the following have consistently shown to be clinically beneficial for patients with GBS?
   A. plasma exchange
   B. intravenous immune globulin administration
   C. steroid administration
   D. none of the above

29-15. An abnormal thymus gland is associated with which of the following?
   A. MG
   B. GBS
   C. porphyria
   D. multiple sclerosis

29-16. Which of the following is true concerning the Tensilon test?
   A. in myasthenic crisis, muscle strength will improve
   B. in cholinergic crisis, muscle strength will deteriorate
   C. both of the above
   D. none of the above

29-17. Which of the following is typically an ascending paralysis?
   A. ALS
   B. GBS
   C. MG
   D. Lambert-Eaton myasthenic syndrome

29-18. Which of the following is true concerning Duchenne's muscular dystrophy?
   A. onset is late in life
   B. it is an autosomal recessive trait
   C. its main physiologic problem is muscle contracture
   D. it occurs in males much more frequently than females

29-19. All of the following are signs of a paralyzed diaphragm except:
   A. inward motion of the abdomen during inspiration
   B. dyspnea in the supine position
   C. cephalad movement during the sniff test
   D. decreased expiratory pressures

29-20. Patients with GBS would most likely have a drop in which of the following **first**?
   A. inspiratory capacity
   B. expiratory pressures
   C. inspiratory pressures
   D. PaO_2

30

Infectious Disease Aspects of Respiratory Therapy

Microbes are ubiquitous (found everywhere). Many microbes are beneficial to mankind and others are not. Our goal is not to eliminate all microorganisms but to prevent patients from becoming contaminated with microbes that may be harmful to them. Proper handwashing, equipment cleaning techniques, and adherence to proper infection control guidelines will help to meet our goal. Chapter 30 in *Respiratory Care* discusses important aspects of infection control.

REVIEW QUESTIONS

30-1. Each of the following is a prokaryote except:
   A. bacteria
   B. chlamydia
   C. rickettsiae
   D. fungi

30-2. The protein coat surrounding the central core of a virus is called:
   A. a spore
   B. a capsid
   C. an anaerobe
   D. an adhesin

30-3. Obligate intracellular parasites include each of the following except:
   A. chlamydia
   B. mycobacteria
   C. rickettsiae
   D. viruses

30-4. The first line of defense against microbes is which of the following?
   A. passive immunity
   B. antibiotics
   C. the skin
   D. a cough

30-5. Large numbers of which of the following cells indicate sputum contaminated with oropharyngeal secretions?
   A. squamous epithelial cells
   B. mycobacteria
   C. *H. capsulatum*
   D. Legionella

30-6. Handwashing should occur:
   A. before working with patients
   B. after working with patients
   C. before and after working with patients
   D. only if gloves are not used

30-7. Transmission of HIV has been linked to all of the following except:
   A. blood
   B. semen
   C. vaginal secretions
   D. urine

30-8. A more specific antibody test used to confirm infection with HIV is the:
   A. enzyme immunoassay
   B. Western blot
   C. gram stain
   D. serum IgG analysis

30-9. To "guarantee" that a piece of equipment is sterilized, which of the following processes can be used?
   A. ethylene oxide
   B. quaternary ammonium compounds
   C. phenols
   D. all of the above

30-10. Approximately half of all epidemics of nosocomial blood stream infections are related to:
   A. intravascular catheters
   B. Foley catheters
   C. oral endotracheal tubes
   D. tracheostomy tubes

31

Interstitial Lung Disease

CASE STUDIES

Case Study 1

W. T. was a very pleasant 48-year-old man who came to the hospital on 1/28/96. He complained of flu-like symptoms, which he had for the past week. These symptoms included upset stomach, myalgia (muscle aches), loss of appetite, low-grade fever and night chills, diarrhea, lethargy (a washed out feeling), and a cough with bloody sputum production.

W. T.'s medical history was significant. He suffered from tobacco abuse from 1960 to present, with a 35+ pack/year smoking history. He suffered from alcoholism from 1970 to 1992 but denied drinking after that time. He had a ruptured appendix in 1992, which lead to peritonitis and the need for a ileostomy. This was eventually corrected.

He had been suffering from chronic diarrhea, malabsorption syndrome, and pancreatic insufficiency secondary to recurrent pancreatitis (since 1987) secondary to alcoholism. In February 1995, he was placed on total parenteral nutrition (TPN). After several weeks of treatment, he gained weight, going from 135 pounds to 146 pounds. At this point, TPN was discontinued and he was placed on oral supplements and pancreatic enzymes.

In April of 1995, he fell and dislocated his shoulder. In October of 1995, he had bowel surgery for a small bowel obstruction. Following his surgery, a right lower lobe density was seen on chest radiograph. This was thought to represent

atelectasis. W. T.'s last admission was in November 1995, when he presented to the hospital in acute renal failure (ARF) secondary to decreased free water absorption. His blood urea nitrogen (BUN) was 119 mg/dL (normal, 10 to 20), creatine 6.8 mg/dL (normal, 1.0), and potassium 6.7 mEq/L (normal, 3.5 to 5). This was rapidly corrected with intravenous hydration and W. T. was discharged in a few days, seemingly recovered.

W. T.'s medical condition seemed to have stabilized until 2 months after his episode of ARF when he presented to the hospital with flu-like symptoms on 1/28/96. Because of his reported symptoms, W. T. was placed in respiratory isolation in a negative flow room. At this time he denied shortness of breath (SOB) and did not require supplemental oxygen. A chest radiograph revealed a right upper lobe interstitial process with the presence of a cavity. On 1/30/96, sputum cultures were positive for aspergillus. On 1/30/96, a bronchoscopy was performed and confirmed a necrotizing aspergillus pneumonia. Treatment was begun with Amphotericin and other broad-spectrum antibiotics. Nasal oxygen was started to keep $SpO_2 > 93\%$. W. T. showed slight improvement for a few days but on 2/4/96 he became very SOB. An ABG revealed a pH of 7.44, $PaCO_2$ of 26 mmHg, PaO_2 of 57 mmHg, Sat of 87%, and a HCO_3 of 18 mM/L on a nonrebreathing mask. A chest radiograph revealed spread of the infection to the total right lung. At this point, W. T. was transferred to the intensive care unit. Following this acute episode, W. T. again showed improvement. He continued to receive his routine respiratory treatments and was able to use nasal cannula at 5 L/min to keep his $SpO_2 > 93\%$. His temperature, however, remained at 102°F. On 2/11/96, following demonstration by radiograph that increased fluid had collected in the right pleural space, a diagnostic thoracentesis was attempted. No fluid was aspirated. On 2/12/96, chest radiograph demonstrated spread of the process to the left lung as well. Although the radiographic picture was worsening, the patient stated he felt better.

On 2/16/96, W. T. developed severe respiratory distress. He was intubated and placed on mechanical ventilation; PC (pressure control) of 24 cmH_2O, frequency of 23, V_T of 600 to 700 mL, PEEP of +5 cmH_2O, and FIO_2 of 80%. An arterial blood gas (ABG) test revealed a pH of 7.42, $PaCO_2$ of 43 mmHg, PaO_2 of 65 mmHg, and an SaO_2 of 92%. Over the next days, W. T. continued to deteriorate. PC was increased to 30 to 35 cmH_2O, VE was greater than 20 L/min, positive end-expiratory pressure (PEEP) was 7 to 11 cmH_2O, and FIO_2 was at 100%. Owing to the extent of lung involvement, only the left upper lobe appeared to be involved in gas exchange. Even with the ventilatory support mentioned above, pH values ranged from 7.13 to 7.25, $PaCO_2$ ranged from 70 to 103 mmHg, and the PaO_2 was in the 50s. W. T. died on 2/25/96 owing to a severe necrotizing aspergillus pneumonia, renal failure, and other medical complications.

Case Study 2

J. R. is a 73-year-old man who presented with increased hand, wrist, and shoulder pain 2 years ago. Diagnosed as having rheumatoid arthritis, he was started on low-dose prednisone, 3 mg/day, and methotrexate, 2.5 mg 3 times/week. Over the course of the following year, his medications were adjusted slightly but yielded only mild relief from his symptoms. A chest radiograph after 1 year of treatment was interpreted as "normal." At the end of 2 years of therapy, a repeat chest radiograph was obtained. The radiograph demonstrated a diffuse interstitial infiltrate with a bilateral reticulonodular pattern, which was more prominent in the right lung field. A computed tomography scan was performed and showed small nodular densities most evident in the upper lobes. Owing to concern that the infiltrate may be drug-induced, methotrexate was discontinued, prednisone was increased to 10 mg/day, and J. R. was scheduled for a pulmonary consult.

On evaluation, J. R. was found to be a well-developed but slightly overweight male with an abnormal chest radiograph but in no apparent distress. His joint pain had gotten worse since the methotrexate was discontinued. He had bilateral basilar crackles but otherwise clear breath sounds. He complained of mild dyspnea on exertion, especially climbing stairs, and an occasional wheeze at night. He had no cough, expectoration, or hemoptysis. His blood pressure was 130/80, and other than the mentioned findings, his physical examination was unremarkable. He has a 120 pack/year smoking history but stopped smoking 18 years ago. He also worked in a foundry (shipping and receiving) for 42 years, but still had considerable exposure to dust. He does not have any contact with birds. A pulmonary function test revealed a combined mild restrictive and obstructive defect with a mildly reduced diffusion capacity. There was no improvement with the administration of a bronchodilator. Forced vital capacity (FVC) = 2.23 L (77%), forced expiratory volume in 1 second (FEV_1) = 1.66 L (75%), FEV_1% = 74%, FEF_{25-75} = 1.14 L/sec (36%), PF = 7.92 L/sec (120%), D_LCO = 16.9 mL/min/mmHg (69%). An ABG and routine laboratory studies were normal. A low level exercise study to check for oxygen desaturation was not conducted at this time.

Impressions from the findings included work-related silicosis, rheumatoid lung disease, or drug-induced (methotrexate) lung disease. Silicosis is highly suspected because of (1) a long history of foundry work, (2) a relatively asymptomatic state, and (3) the presence of radiographic abnormalities on previous radiographs. (The radiographs from the previous year were re-evaluated, and the reticulonodular pattern was definitely present). J. R. is being closely observed and will have repeat radiographs and PFTs in 3 months.

REVIEW QUESTIONS

31-1. Each of the following are part of the lung interstitium except:
  A. lymphatics
  B. connective tissue
  C. alveolar space
  D. capillaries

31-2. Common features of interstitial lung disease (ILD) include each of the following except:
  A. progressive dyspnea
  B. hypercarbia
  C. restrictive pulmonary dysfunction
  D. exercise-induced hypoxemia

31-3. The first indicator of ILD in its early stages is often:
  A. a persistent cough
  B. dyspnea
  C. low-grade fever
  D. an incidental chest radiograph

31-4. The end stage of many forms of ILD is often represented by:
  A. emphysema
  B. fibrosis
  C. bronchiectasis
  D. chronic obstructive pulmonary disease

31-5. Which of the following are classified as extrinsic causes of ILD?
  A. administration of chemotherapeutic agents
  B. scleroderma
  C. rheumatoid arthritis
  D. all of the above

31-6. Which of the following are possible reasons why some individuals are more likely to develop ILD than others?
  A. individual susceptibility
  B. integrity of the immune system
  C. genetic predisposition
  D. all of the above

31-7. Which of the following techniques best allows diagnosis of the various types of ILD?
  A. chest radiograph
  B. high-resolution computed tomography
  C. magnetic resonance imaging
  D. radionuclide imaging

31-8. The most common cause of ILD in western countries is:
  A. sarcoidosis
  B. drug induced
  C. lung transplantation
  D. idiopathic pulmonary fibrosis

31-9. The main therapy for patients with advancing idiopathic pulmonary fibrosis is:
  A. oxygen
  B. corticosteroids
  C. immunosuppressive drugs
  D. anti-inflammatory agents

31-10. Which of the following is most reliable for diagnosis of sarcoidosis?
A. serologic tests
B. skin anergy tests
C. serum angiotensin converting enzyme levels
D. biopsy of involved organs

31-11. The most important aspect of managing acute hypersensitivity pneumonitis is:
A. the use of antimicrobial agents
B. patient education
C. the use of anti-inflammatory agents
D. the use of bronchodilators

31-12. Nonpulmonary disorders causing ILD include each of the following except:
A. rheumatoid arthritis
B. lupus erythematosus
C. silicosis
D. scleroderma

31-13. ILD usually results in all of the following pulmonary function changes except:
A. decreased D_LCO
B. increased functional residual capacity
C. decreased vital capacity
D. no change in flow rates

31-14. The drug most commonly reported to produce pulmonary abnormalities is:
A. Busulfan (chemotherapeutic)
B. Nitrofurantoin (antibiotic)
C. aspirated oils
D. Gold salts

31-15. Oxygen toxicity can be avoided if the FiO_2 is kept below what maximum concentration?
A. 40%
B. 50%
C. 60%
D. 70%

32

Work-Related, Environmentally Caused, and Self-Induced Pulmonary Disorders

REVIEW QUESTIONS

32-1. MSDS is:
   A. an interstitial lung disease
   B. a subcommittee of OSHA
   C. an ad hoc committee of NIOSH
   D. an information sheet on hazardous substances

32-2. Development of mesothelioma is caused by exposure to:
   A. asbestos fibers
   B. toxic gases
   C. silicon
   D. tuberculosis

32-3. A characteristic "egg shell" classification of the hilar lymph nodes may be observed in:
   A. asbestosis
   B. silicosis
   C. tuberculosis
   D. occupational asthma

32-4. Tuberculosis transmission is classified as:
   A. vector transmission
   B. airborne
   C. vehicle transmission
   D. direct contact

32-5. Most authors recommend a four-drug regimen for tuberculosis treatment in areas where drug resistance is increased. Each of the following is included except:
   A. isoniazid
   B. streptomycin

   C. amphotericin B
   D. rifampin

32-6. Useful clinical data for positive diagnosis of occupational asthma include each of the following except:
   A. decreased spirometry values after exposure
   B. decreased peak flow following exposure
   C. a diary of increased symptoms with exposure
   D. a negative methacholine test

32-7. COHb levels in normal urban settings do not exceed which of the following levels?
   A. 1%
   B. 2.5%
   C. 4.8%
   D. 6.4%

32-8. One of the most common causes of death in patients admitted with burns is:
   A. dehydration
   B. congestive heart failure
   C. pneumothorax
   D. infections

32-9. Early intubation in the burn patient should be considered in all of the following situations except:
   A. greater than 40% cutaneous burn injury
   B. presence of mucosal burns
   C. singed facial hair with less than 10% cutaneous burn
   D. presence of a carbonaceous material in the airway

32-10. Early tracheotomy should be avoided in burn patients owing to which of the following:
   A. high risk of serious bleeding
   B. high risk if pneumothorax
   C. high risk of aspiration
   D. high risk if secondary infection

32-11. A common complication of high minute ventilation is the development of auto-PEEP. All of the following may help decrease auto-PEEP levels except:
   A. use of IMV
   B. use of low I:E ratio ventilation
   C. use of large tidal volumes
   D. allowing permissive hypercapnia

32-12. Approximately what percent of the current smokers state that they want to quit smoking and have tried at least once?
   A. 20%
   B. 35%
   C. 50%
   D. 65%

32-13. Each of the following is a symptom of nicotine withdrawal except:
   A. weight loss
   B. craving for tobacco
   C. bradycardia
   D. restlessness

33

Acute Respiratory Failure

CASE STUDY

E. S. is a 59-year-old man with chronic obstructive pulmonary disease (COPD). He had been on home oxygen therapy at 1 L/min for 3 years and doing rather well. Although using continuous oxygen via nasal cannula, E. S. continued to smoke cigarettes. In August, while visiting family members out of his home area, E. S. was involved in a motor vehicle accident (MVA). He had been trying to manipulate his oxygen while lighting a cigarette. E. S. was taken to the local community hospital via ambulance and was admitted to the emergency department. Evaluation revealed a well-developed male with a bump on his head and a bruised arm and hip. Injuries appeared minor, radiographs revealed no broken bones, and other findings were unremarkable. After consulting with family members, it was decided that E. S. would be admitted overnight for observation and released in the morning. Being out of state, the only history available was that which the family and E. S. were able to provide. An arterial blood gas (ABG) study was not obtained at the time of admission.

E. S. was admitted to a general floor and placed on 1 L/min nasal cannula. That evening, E. S. had no complaints, his vital signs were stable, and he had a restful evening. Little was noted during the night shift except that the patient slept peacefully. In the morning, the nurses could not arouse E. S. An ABG was obtained and it was noted that the oxygen setting was on 2 L/min. The results of the ABG were as follows: pH = 7.06, $PaCO_2$ = 149 mmHg, PaO_2 = 68 mmHg, O_2Sat = 83%, and

HCO_3 = 48 mEq/L. The attending physician was notified, and E. S. was intubated and placed on mechanical ventilation. Within a short time, E. S. was alert and awake and was able to be extubated without further complications.

Questions to consider (answers appear in Answer Key):

1. What is the ABG interpretation?
2. Why did E. S. go into acute respiratory failure?
3. What FIO_2 was E. S. receiving while on the 2 L/min?
4. At a PaO_2 of 68 mmHg, the O_2Sat should have been close to 95%. Why was it only 83%?
5. What was the target value for $PaCO_2$ when E. S. was placed on mechanical ventilation?

REVIEW QUESTIONS

33-1. Which of the following are correct concerning acute respiratory failure (ARF)?
  A. it is a dysfunction of the respiratory system leading to hypercarbia
  B. it is a dysfunction of the respiratory system leading to a critical shortage of oxygen delivery to the tissues
  C. ARF may result in an altered mental status
  D. all of the above
33-2. Each of the following are clinically significant causes of hypoxemia except:
  A. hypoventilation
  B. $\dot{V}/\dot{Q}$ mismatch
  C. diffusion impairment
  D. right-to-left shunt
33-3. In the upright position, an individual will have a greater amount of his or her ventilation go to which portion of the lung?
  A. apex
  B. middle
  C. base
  D. posterior
33-4. In the upright position, an individual will have a greater amount of their circulation go to which portion of the lung?
  A. apex
  B. middle
  C. base
  D. posterior
33-5. The $\dot{V}/\dot{Q}$ ratio is highest in which area of the lung?
  A. apex
  B. middle
  C. base
  D. posterior
33-6. A pulmonary embolus causes hypoxemia primarily because of:
  A. shunt

Copyright © 1997, Lippincott–Raven Publishers, Instructor's Manual to Accompany Burton, Hodgkin, Ward: Respiratory Care: A Guide to Clinical Practice, 4th edition

B. $\dot{V}/\dot{Q}$ mismatch
C. hypoventilation
D. diffusion defect

33-7. Atelectasis causes hypoxemia primarily because of:
    A. shunt
    B. $\dot{V}/\dot{Q}$ mismatch
    C. hypoventilation
    D. diffusion defect

33-8. A patient with hypoxemia but with a normal A-a gradient is most likely suffering from hypoxemia because of:
    A. shunt
    B. $\dot{V}/\dot{Q}$ mismatch
    C. hypoventilation
    D. diffusion defect

33-9. Paradoxical motion of the thorax (out) and abdomen (in), in a spontaneously breathing patient, often indicates:
    A. diaphragm weakness
    B. decreased central drive to breathe
    C. respiratory alkalosis
    D. flail chest

33-10. The immediate treatment of acute hypoxemia should involve oxygen administration to achieve a minimum hemoglobin saturation of what percent?
    A. 88%
    B. 90%
    C. 93%
    D. 95%

33-11. Oxygenation of a patient on mechanical ventilation has been shown to be enhanced by which of the following flow patterns?
    A. accelerating
    B. decelerating
    C. square
    D. constant

33-12. The gold standard for diagnosis of a pulmonary embolus is:
    A. an ABG
    B. the pulmonary angiogram

C. the $\dot{V}/\dot{Q}$ scan
D. impedance plethysmography

33-13. To reduce the risk of barotrauma, which of the following should be considered?
    A. keep PEEP above the inflection point pressure
    B. use small tidal volumes
    C. keep peak airway pressure less than 35 cmH_2O
    D. all of the above

33-14. The use of Narcan is appropriate in which of the following causes of type II respiratory failure?
    A. use of barbiturates
    B. alcohol intoxication
    C. intracranial hemorrhage
    D. use of morphine

33-15. An asthmatic in moderated distress with normal blood gases in the emergency department should be:
    A. sent home with prn bronchodilator use
    B. monitored with prn bronchodilator use
    C. treated aggressively with bronchodilators
    D. intubated and placed on mechanical ventilation

33-16. The cornerstone of immediate therapy for obstructive lung disease is:
    A. inhaled beta agonists
    B. inhaled anticholinergic agents
    C. systemic theophylline
    D. systemic corticosteroids

33-17. Permissive hypercapnia would most likely benefit a patient with which of the following?
    A. COPD
    B. asthma
    C. massive obesity
    D. kyphoscoliosis

34

Acute or Adult Respiratory Distress Syndrome

CASE STUDY

B. H. is a 67-year-old woman who was diagnosed with breast cancer in 1980. This had been surgically treated, and since then she had been doing fine. In January 1996, she experienced a left-sided brain stroke. She recovered from this quite well, and in early November at a routine medical checkup stated that she had good functional status and was enjoying life.

Two weeks later, in mid November, B. H. presented in the emergency department with left-sided abdominal pain, hypotension, and shortness of breath. B. H. said that she had been feeling this way for 2 days and that she was not voiding very much. Urinalysis, blood cultures, complete blood count, and an arterial blood gas (ABG) test were performed. The ABG revealed a metabolic acidosis with mild hypoxemia. B. H. was started on 2 L/min nasal cannula and admitted with a suspected urinary tract infection (UTI) and acute renal failure (ARF). B. H.'s blood pressure remained unstable, and her condition began to deteriorate. Blood cultures revealed a septicemia, and within 48 hours of admission, B. H. was intubated and placed on mechanical ventilation. She was initially placed on volume control ventilation; f = 12 b/min, V_T = 700 mL, FIO_2 – 50%, and PEEP of +5 cmH_2O. ABGs were as follows: pH = 7.29, $PaCO_2$ = 26 mmHg, and PaO_2 = 118 mmHg. Within 12 hours of intubation, her compliance began to deteriorate, and the peak in-

spiratory pressure (PIP) began to climb. At this point, the settings were changed to pressure control ventilation to help prevent pressure damage to the lungs. Typical settings for the next 3 days were as follows: f = 16 to 20 b/min, PIP = 33 to 37 cmH_2O, FIO_2 = 80% to 100%, and PEEP of 10 to 13 cmH_2O. Her compliance ranged from 16 to 22 mL/cmH_2O. A typical ABG during this time revealed a pH of 7.38, $PaCO_2$ of 39 mmHg, and PaO_2 of 57 mmHg. Her blood pressure remained low and very unstable, and there were signs of development of anoxic encephalopathy. Four days following intubation, her respiratory system took a turn for the better, and she was able to be weaned to 50% oxygen and +8 of PEEP. The next day, she was able to be weaned to 30% oxygen and +5 of PEEP.

Although B. H.'s respiratory system improved, her cardiac, neurologic, and overall clinical condition did not. Two weeks following admission, B. H. expired.

REVIEW QUESTIONS

34-1. Define ARDS: _____

_____

_____

_____

34-2. List the three phases of the pathological process of ARDS: _____

_____

_____

_____

34-3. Which of the following is not characteristic of ARDS?
   A. alveolar edema
   B. increased shunt
   C. increased compliance
   D. increased dead space

34-4. Respiratory system abnormalities seen in ARDS include each of the following except:
   A. pulmonary hypotension
   B. right ventricular failure
   C. deranged respiratory drive
   D. respiratory muscle fatigue

34-5. Which of the following is a major antioxidant found in the epithelial lining cells?
   A. guanylyl cyclase
   B. peroxynitrite
   C. reduced glutathione

D. cyclooxygenase

34-6. Which of the following best describes nitric oxide?
A. anti-inflammatory agent
B. vasodilator
C. bronchodilator
D. respiratory stimulant

34-7. Which of the following strategies has clearly been shown to alter the development of ARDS?
A. use of PEEP
B. gut sterilization
C. nutritional support
D. none of the above

34-8. It has been suggested that maximal alveolar pressures be kept below what levels?
A. <45 cmH$_2$O
B. <40 cmH$_2$O
C. <35 cmH$_2$O
D. <30 cmH$_2$O

34-9. Maximal alveolar pressures are estimated by measuring which of the following?
A. peak airway pressure
B. plateau pressure
C. mean airway pressure
D. PEEP level

34-10. Each of the following are predictors of increased mortality risk in ARDS except:
A. initial gas exchange severity
B. sepsis syndrome
C. evidence of tissue hypoxia
D. advanced age

34-11. Which of the following is true concerning ARDS?
A. death is often caused by respiratory failure
B. inadequate respiratory support capabilities are a major cause of mortality
C. long-term prognosis appears good if the patient survives the initial episode of ARDS
D. pulmonary function tests in ARDS survivors show poor return of function

35

Respiratory Care in the Coronary Care Unit

CASE STUDIES

Case Study 1

M. T. is a 158-lb, 61-year-old, retired man who had a routine physical in July 1996. ECG changes were noted and a Thallium stress test was scheduled. During the stress test, he was able to exercise for 9 minutes and 22 seconds without chest pain, but the test was positive for changes significant for ischemia. An echo was performed and demonstrated anteroapical ischemia. A cardiac catheterization was recommended.

M. T. has had hyperlipidemia, tobacco abuse for 50 years, and a strong family history for heart disease (his father died at age 48 years of a myocardial infarction). He has had no symptoms of chest pain or respiratory distress.

The following laboratory tests were obtained before the catheterization: white blood cell count $10.4 \times 10^3/mm^3$, red blood cell count $5.0 \times 10^6/mm^3$, platelets $188 \times 10^3/mm^3$, hemoglobin 16.2 g/dL, hematocrit 45.9 %, blood urea nitrogen 21 mg/dL, creatine 0.8 mg/dL, Na 142 mEq/L, K 4.3 mEq/L, glucose 101 mg/dL, prothrombin 11.2 seconds, and partial thromblastin time 25.1 seconds. His triglycerides were high at 278 mg/dL, cholesterol 216 mg/dL, high-density lipoprotein 40 mg/dL, low-density lipoprotein 120 mg/dL. His chest radiograph was within normal limits.

In early August, a left heart catheterization using the right femoral technique was performed. M. T. had a normal left ventricle with an esti-

mated ejection fraction of 60%. On examination of the coronary arteries, the left circumflex (LCX) was 80% occluded and the right coronary artery (RCA) was 60% to 70% occluded. A percutaneous transluminal coronary angioplasty (PTCA) with a stent implantation in the LCX was recommended. This would be followed by stress tests to assess the severity of disease in the RCA. If flow limitations would be noted, a stent would be placed in the RCA also. M. T. went home to discuss this with his family and 2 days later contacted the cardiologist to schedule the procedure.

Four days before the PTCA, M. T. began taking Ticlid. This drug helps assure that the platelets will not adhere to the stent. In late August, M. T was admitted to the hospital for the first time in his life. A successful PTCA with stent insertion was performed. M. T. tolerated the procedure well, but did have some chest pain and ECG changes with the balloon inflation. He was admitted to the coronary unit overnight and the next day discharged with the following instructions. There should be no heavy lifting for 48 hours. Maintain a low-sodium, low-fat diet. Have a repeat CBC in 2 weeks and a Thallium stress test in 1 month. He was to take 1 aspirin/day, 5 mg of Norvasc/day to prevent hypertension, and Ticlid at 250 mg twice a day for 1 month.

Follow-up showed that M. T. did not require an RCA stent, and he continues to be asymptomatic. He will be observed closely for future changes that may occur.

Case Study 2

J. S. is a 66-year-old male truck driver who was unable to work because of chest discomfort. He had a Thallium stress test in April 1996, and it was markedly abnormal with the patient experiencing chest pain 2.5 minutes into the test. A cardiac catheterization was recommended, but J. S. wanted to try medical treatment first. This was not successful, and since he could not work, he agreed to the catheterization.

Laboratory tests were normal except for cholesterol, which was mildly elevated. J. S. does have a 20-year history of diabetes, but refused to use insulin for fear of losing his job. He has a 100 pack/year smoking history and is 80 lb over his ideal body weight.

In late July, a cardiac catheterization was performed. The right femoral artery catheterization showed the left anterior descending (LAD) to be 95% occluded. The diagonal was 90% occluded, obtuse marginal 1 (OM1) was 70% occluded, and the OM2 90% occluded. The right coronary artery had minimal disease, and the left ventricle was normal with an estimated ejection fraction of 65%. J. S. was found to have severe CAD and coronary artery bypass grafts were recommended for the LAD, diagonal, OM1, and OM2. J. S. was discharged and scheduled for surgery.

Before surgery, a pulmonary function test and arterial blood gas (ABG) test were performed on J. S. as an outpatient. The ABG was normal and the PFT showed a mild obstructive pattern. J. S. was admitted mid August for his surgery. During surgery Versed, Fentanyl, and Diprivan were used to maintain anesthesia. Two grafts were done. The left internal mammary artery was grafted onto the LAD, and a saphenous vein from the right thigh was used to bypass the OM1. The OM2 was too small to bypass. J. S. was weaned from the bypass machine without the aid of inotropic support. Chest tubes were inserted for drainage. Protamine was given to reverse the heparinization that was necessary for the bypass machine. J. S. was admitted to the intensive care unit (ICU) at 6 PM. He was set up on a Star ventilator on synchronized intermittent mechanical ventilation (SIMV) rate of 12/min, V_T of 900 mL, 100% oxygen, +5 positive end-expiratory pressure (PEEP), and pressure support (PS) of +8 cmH$_2$O. His ABG on these settings were, pH 7.37, PaCO$_2$ 41 mmHg, and PaO$_2$ 88 mmHg. A chest radiograph showed normal postoperative atelectatic changes at the left base and all tubes in their proper positions. At 7:10 PM, four puffs of albuterol Q4 were given for wheezing. A small amount of yellow sputum was being suctioned. Since only minimal sedation was being given, J. S. was awake and following commands by 7:40 PM. Because J. S. was improving, at 8:25 PM the FiO$_2$ was decreased to 60% and the SIMV to 6/min. Following an ABG, spontaneous breathing parameters were done. His frequency was 24/min, V_T was 550 mL, maximum inspiratory pressure (MIP) was −53 cmH$_2$O, and his VC was 1.2 L. J. S. was then placed on PS mode of ventilation at +8 cmH$_2$O with an FiO$_2$ of 60% and PEEP of +5 cmH$_2$O. An ABG revealed a pH of 7.31, PaCO$_2$ of 40 mmHg, and a PaO$_2$ of 131 mmHg. At 9:45, 3 hours and 45 minutes after arriving in the ICU, J. S. was extubated and placed on 6 L/min nasal cannula. A post-extubation ABG showed a pH of 7.33, PaCO$_2$ of 38 mmHg, and a PaO$_2$ of 94 mmHg. He was immediately started on incentive spirometry (ISB), achieving 1.5 L. His lungs were clear and he had a strong cough. Within the first 5 hours in the ICU, J. S. received albumin, dopamine, insulin, nitroglycerine, and 3 amps of bicarb. His intake was 2203 mL, and his output was 2755 mL. Chest tube drainage totalled 640 mL. His hemodynamic measurements were as follows: pulmonary capillary wedge pressure 6 to 10 mmHg, CO 7.7 to 9.6 L, MAP 58 to 91 mmHg, and SvO$_2$ 63% to 79%.

The morning chest radiograph, postoperative day 1 (POD 1), showed less atelectasis at the left base, but a small effusion was still present. The left chest tube was still in place with a small amount of subcutaneous air noted over the left pectoralis muscle. His ECG revealed a right bundle branch block. He achieved 1.25 L with his ISB and his SpO$_2$ was 97% on 5 L/min. His peak flows were 270 L/min and did not improve with bronchodilators, so they were changed to prn. After removal of the pulmonary artery catheter, J. S. was transferred out of the unit. On POD 2, the Foley catheter was removed. Oxygen was decreased to maintain SpO$_2$ > 92%. An air leak was still present, so suction was maintained on the chest tube. Auscultation revealed occasional crackles.

On POD 3, his oxygen flow was at 1.5 L/min, and there was no air leak in the chest tube, so it was removed. All incisions were healing well. On POD 4, pacer wires were removed and J. S. attended an instructional discharge class. He was encouraged to attend an outpatient healthy heart eating class. He was also given instruction concerning his diabetes before discharge. J. S. was prescribed the following medications: Darvocet prn for pain, Ascriptin, Glucophage, and Glyburide. A home health agency was contacted for follow-up care in the home.

REVIEW QUESTIONS

35-1. Cardiovascular disease accounts for approximately how many deaths annually in the United States?
A. 100,000
B. 500,000
C. 1,000,000
D. 5,000,000

35-2. Cardiac arrest victims are most often in which of the following dysrhythmias?
A. V-fib
B. V-tach
C. 2° block
D. 3° block

35-3. Each of the following are risk factors for development of CAD except:
A. hypotension
B. male gender
C. increased age
D. family history of CAD

35-4. The classic symptom of myocardial ischemia is:
A. angina pectoris
B. diaphoresis
C. vertigo
D. dyspnea

35-5. Which of the following ECG changes is seen with myocardial infarction?
A. P-R interval elongation
B. S-wave inversion
C. T-wave spiking
D. S-T segment elevation

35-6. Technetium Tc 99m can be used to assess all of the following except:
A. whether an infarct has occurred
B. to localize the area of infarct
C. to establish the size of an infarct
D. ventricular wall motion

35-7. The standard for defining coronary artery anatomy is the:
A. MUGA scan
B. coronary angiography
C. Thallium scan
D. echocardiography

35-8. Morphine is often used to relieve pain and anxiety in patients with myocardial infarctions. All of the following may be side effects of morphine except:
   A. hypotension
   B. tachypnea
   C. bradycardia
   D. nausea

35-9. Nitrates have each of the following effects except:
   A. to increase coronary artery blood flow
   B. to increase preload
   C. to decrease afterload
   D. to decrease oxygen demand

35-10. Treatment with thrombolytic agents for coronary occlusion:
   A. is most beneficial if given within several hours
   B. is mediated by the fibrinolytic system
   C. has been shown to improve mortality rates compared with placebo
   D. all of the above

35-11. The major risk of thrombolytic therapy is:
   A. bleeding
   B. coronary re-occlusion
   C. sudden death
   D. pulmonary thrombus formation

36

Respiratory Care of the Surgical Patient

CASE STUDY

M. D. is a 40-year-old man who was admitted in November with multiple stab wounds but in stable condition. His initial blood pressure was 112/67, heart rate was 109, and SpO_2 was 99%. On examination, a 3-cm substernal wound was found with smooth borders, which was draining venous blood. A portable chest radiograph revealed a dilated cardiac silhouette. His blood gas revealed a pH of 7.05, $PaCO_2$ of 46 mmHg, PaO_2 of 92 mmHg, O_2Sat of 92%, and HCO_3 of 13 mEq/L on a non-rebreathing mask. The severe acidosis was most likely caused by hypoxia and lactic acid production before treatment. The patient was taken to the operating room for exploratory laparotomy and midline sternotomy. The sternotomy revealed a pericardial blood clot that was evacuated. There was also a right ventricular laceration that was repaired. Other findings were amazingly unremarkable. A mediastinal chest tube remained in place following surgery.

The patient was then transferred to the intensive care unit and placed on volume ventilation. Initially, ventilating pressures were in the 40 cmH_2O range, and his compliance was in the low 20s. It was decided to place the patient on the pressure control mode to hopefully prevent lung injury caused by the high peak and plateau pressures. On a frequency of 12 b/min, peak inspiratory pressure (PIP) of 25 cmH_2O, Ti of 1.25 sec, FIO_2 of 50%, and a positive end-expiratory pressure (PEEP) of +10 cmH_2O, his arterial blood gases (ABGs) were pH = 7.24, $PaCO_2$ = 44 mmHg, PaO_2 = 63 mmHg, O_2Sat = 89%, and HCO_3 19 mEq/L.

Following this ABG, PEEP was increased to 15 cm H_2O. Soon afterwards, his compliance improved to 40 mL/cmH_2O, and his PaO_2 increased to 138 mmHg. M. D. continued to improve, FIO_2 was decreased, PEEP was decreased, and PIP was decreased as compliance and tidal volume increased. On postoperative day 1, M. D. was alert, had a chest radiograph within normal limits, was placed on pressure support of +8, and was extubated. On postoperative day 2, M. D. continued to improve, was inhaling over 2 L on the incentive spirometer, and was transferred out of the intensive care unit.

REVIEW QUESTIONS

36-1. Incisions at which of the following sites would have the most severe effects on the pulmonary system?
   I. upper abdomen
   II. lower abdomen
   III. thorax
   IV. extremity

   A. I and II only
   B. I and III only
   C. II and IV only
   D. II, III, and IV only

36-2. The incidence of postoperative pulmonary complications has been shown to nearly double if the operative time exceeds how many hours?
   A. 1 hour
   B. 3 hours
   C. 5 hours
   D. 7 hours

36-3. A decrease in VC of up to what percent may be well tolerated in most healthy surgical patients?
   A. 25%
   B. 33%
   C. 50%
   D. 75%

36-4. Postoperative decreases in vital capacity are thought to be the result of which of the following?
   A. decreased diaphragmatic muscle function following surgery
   B. respiratory depressant effect of anesthetics
   C. absence of deep breaths
   D. all of the above

36-5. Carbon dioxide retention occurs postoperatively when:
   A. low-but-finite $\dot{V}/\dot{Q}$ is present
   B. $\dot{V}/\dot{Q}$ of zero is present
   C. respiratory depression occurs from use or misuse of narcotics
   D. all of the above

36-6. To show a significant improvement in lung function following smoking cessation, how long should the patient have stopped smoking?
A. 2 weeks
B. 4 weeks
C. 6 weeks
D. 8 weeks

36-7. The most commonly used test that yields the most useful predictive value for development of postoperative complications is:
A. forced vital capacity
B. peak flow
C. functional residual capacity
D. maximum voluntary ventilation

36-8. A forced expiratory volume in 1 second (FEV_1) of less than what value is associated with a significant increase in postoperative morbidity and mortality?
A. <4 L
B. <3 L
C. <2 L
D. <1 L

36-9. Mechanical ventilation sensitivity should be routinely set at:
A. −3 cmH_2O
B. −2 cmH_2O
C. −1 cmH_2O
D. the most sensitive setting while avoiding autocycling

36-10. Which of the following statements are true?
A. there are several "risk-free" anesthetics on the market
B. regional (spinal) techniques often result in decreased postoperative pulmonary complications
C. general anesthesia does not cause diaphragm dysfunction
D. operative time has little effect on postoperative pulmonary complications

36-11. The most common postoperative changes in pulmonary function include each of the following except:
A. severe reduction in surfactant production
B. reduced lung volumes
C. impaired gas exchange
D. abnormal breathing patterns

36-12. Which of the following examinations of the chest is used to assess the presence and quality of air movement?
A. inspection
B. palpation
C. percussion
D. auscultation

Answers

CHAPTER 1

Word Find

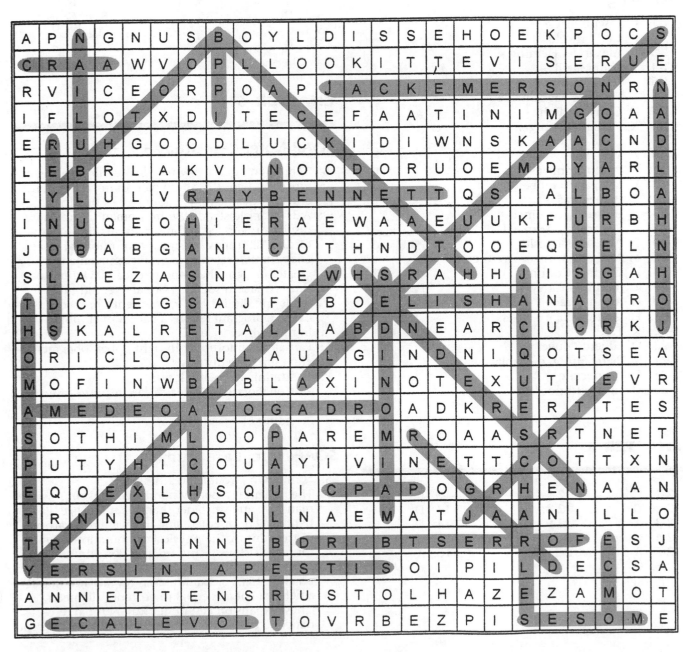

Crossword Puzzle

Down	**Across**
1. Galen	1. Aoyagi
2. Aristotle	2. Pascal
3. Beddoes	3. Hill
4. Clark	4. Erasistratus
5. Servetus	5. Ruben
6. Millikan	6. Boyle
7. Laennec	7. Harvey
8. Hutchinson	8. Hunter
9. Ehrlich	9. Pasteur
10. Waksman	10. Fick
	11. Magnus
	12. Morton
	13. Severinghaus

Matching

1-1.   C   Joseph Black
1-2.   F   Carl Scheele
1-3.   P   Alexander Fleming
1-4.   T   Ivan Magill
1-5.   A   John Dalton
1-6.   N   Florence Nightingale
1-7.   O   Christian Bohr
1-8.   X   William Roentgen
1-9.   R   Clara Barton
1-10. Z VO_2, VCO_2
1-11. I   Philip Drinker
1-12. V   Morgan Campbell
1-13. W   Pythagoras
1-14. H   Leonardo da Vinci
1-15. B   Evangelista Torricelli
1-16. D   Antoine Lavoisier
1-17. M   Anthony van Leeuwenhoek
1-18. L   Gardner Colton
1-19. Y   Joseph Priestley
1-20. G   Alvan Barach
1-21. J   laryngoscope
1-22. K   T.B.
1-23. Q   Eduard Pfluger
1-24. S   Pierre Simon de Laplace
1-25. E   Hippocrates
1-26. U   Sir Arbuthnot Lane

CHAPTER 2

2-1. C	2-7. C	2-12. B
2-2. D	2-8. A	2-13. D
2-3. A	2-9. D	2-14. D
2-4. C	2-10. A	2-15. A
2-5. B	2-11. C	2-16. A
2-6. C		

CHAPTER 4

Review Questions

4-1. C	4-7. B	4-13. A
4-2. B	4-8. C	4-14. D
4-3. D	4-9. D	4-15. C
4-4. A	4-10. A	4-16. A
4-5. B	4-11. C	4-17. B
4-6. C	4-12. D	

CHAPTER 5

5-1. C	5-5. A	5-8. B
5-2. D	5-6. C	5-9. C
5-3. C	5-7. D	5-10. D
5-4. D		

CHAPTER 6

SOAP Note: Case Study 1

S: "About an hour ago while I was carrying a bag of groceries, I got this sharp pain in my right chest and at the same time, I got short of breath."

O: A 35-year-old slender white woman in moderate respiratory distress. Monitor reveals sinus tachycardia. All other vital signs within normal limits. Examination reveals respiratory movement is greater in right chest and tracheal deviation to the left. Breath sounds normal over left lung fields and diminished in the right upper lobe. Chest radiogram reveals a partial pneumothorax in right upper lobe.

A: Partial pneumothorax in right upper lobe; moderate respiratory distress.

P: 1. Administer O_2 at 2 L/min.
    2. Collaborate with health care team to insert chest tube
    3. Admit

SOAP Note: Case Study 2

S: "I'm having trouble breathing."

O: The patient is a poorly nourished, unkempt white man who appears older than his stated age. Patient is alert, oriented, and in severe respiratory distress during the physical examination. Monitor reveals sinus tachycardia at 126/minute, temperature is 38.7°C, respirations 28/min, and blood pressure 154/96. Examination reveals anterior diameter of chest is equal to posterior diameter. Chest expansion is symmetrical. Normal resonance to percussion over most of the chest except the right lower chest, which has decreased resonance. Breath sounds diminished with scattered high-pitched wheezes throughout all lung fields. Fine crackles in right lower lobe. Course rhonchi and bronchial breath sounds in left lower lobe. There is nailbed cyanosis of fingers. No clubbing. +1 pitting edema of ankles. Pulses are +2 in all areas except for dorsalis pedis pulses, which are +1. Chest radiograph shows changes consistent with emphysema. There is consolidation of right lower lobe consistent with lobar pneumonia.

A: Emphysema with right lobar pneumonia; moderate respiratory distress.

P: 1. Obtain ABG
   2. Administer O_2 at 2 L/min; consult with physician and adjust as needed as per ABG
   3. Collaborate with health care team in the administration of bronchodilators, antibiotics, diuretics, and digoxin
   4. Admit

Review Questions

6-4. C	6-10. B	6-16. A
6-5. B	6-11. C	6-17. C
6-6. D	6-12. B	6-18. D
6-7. D	6-13. C	6-19. C
6-8. C	6-14. D	6-20. B
6-9. A	6-15. D	

Matching

6-21. D Crackles
6-22. C Diminished
6-23. F Wheeze
6-24. A Bronchial
6-25. G Pleural friction rub
6-26. H Rhonchi
6-27. E Vesicular
6-28. B Adventitious

CHAPTER 7

Review Questions

7-1. C	7-6. C	7-11. C
7-2. A	7-7. A	7-12. D
7-3. D	7-8. D	7-13. A
7-4. C	7-9. D	7-14. D
7-5. D	7-10. B	

CHAPTER 8

Lung Volumes and Capacities

8-1. V_T = 0.51 L	8-5. IC = 3.47 L
RV = 0.94 L	VC = 4.46 L
FRC = 1.99 L	FRC = 2.0 L
IC = 3.13 L	TLC = 5.47 L
8-2. RV = 1.17 L	8-6. RV = 1.12 L
ERV = 1.2 L	ERV = 1.42 L
IC = 3.4 L	IC = 3.76 L
V_T = 0.53 L	V_T = 0.47 L
8-3. RV = 1.4 L	8-7. TLC = 5.42 L
VC = 4.92 L	ERV = 0.92 L
IC = 3.46 L	IRV = 3.07 L
TLC = 6.32 L	IC = 3.46 L
8-4. TLC = 5.62 L	
ERV = 1.07 L	
IRV = 2.84 L	
IC = 3.41 L	

Volume-Time Curve (approximate values)

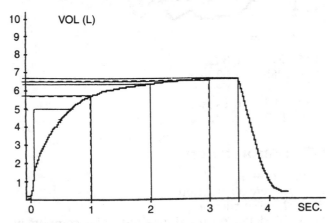

8-8. FVC	6.6 L
8-9. FEV_1	5.7 L
8-10. FEV_1/FVC	86%
8-11. FEV_2	6.3 L
8-12. FEV_3	6.5 L
8-13. FEF_{25-75}	5.5 L/sec
8-14. FET	3.5 sec

Flow-Volume Curve (approximate values)

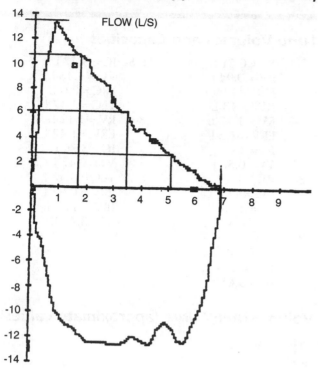

FLOW (L/S)

8-15.	FVC	6.8 L
8-16.	PEF	13.2 L/sec
8-17.	FEF_{25}	10.8 L/sec
8-18.	FEF_{50}	6.1 L/sec
8-19.	FEF_{75}	2.9 L/sec

PFT Interpretation

8-20. Normal
8-21. Severe obstruction
8-22. Mild restriction
8-23. Moderate obstruction, a restrictive component may be present, but it cannot be documented with the limited data given
8-24. Very mild obstruction (early small airway disease)

Lung Volumes and Capacities

8-25.	VC	8-28.	FRC	8-31.	IRV
8-26.	ERV	8-29.	TLC	8-32.	RV
8-27.	TLC	8-30.	ERV		

Review Questions

8-33.	A	8-37.	D	8-41.	C
8-34.	B	8-38.	D	8-42.	B
8-35.	C	8-39.	C	8-43.	C
8-36.	B	8-40.	A	8-44.	A

CHAPTER 9

Partial Pressure and Percent

9-1. $PO_2 = 370$ mmHg, $PN_2 = 370$ mmHg
9-2. $PHe = 546$ mmHg, $PO_2 = 234$ mmHg
9-3. $PT = 620$ mmHg, $FO_2 = 0.113$, $\%O_2 = 11.3\%$, $FCO_2 = 0.048$, $\%CO_2 = 4.8\%$ $FN_2 = 0.839$, $\%N_2 = 83.9\%$
9-4. $PO_2 = 760$ mmHg

PIO_2 and PAO_2

	PIO_2	PAO_2
9-5.	214 mmHg	164 mmHg
9-6.	713 mmHg	673 mmHg
9-7.	214 mmHg	114 mmHg
9-8.	125 mmHg	50 mmHg
9-9.	297 mmHg	247 mmHg
9-10.	120 mmHg	95 mmHg
9-11.	150 mmHg	125 mmHg
9-12.	499 mmHg	449 mmHg

a/A Ratio and A-a Gradient

	A-a grad	a/A ratio
9-13.	44 mmHg	0.73
9-14.	123 mmHg	0.82
9-15.	54 mmHg	0.53
9-16.	5 mmHg	0.90
9-17.	47 mmHg	0.81
9-18.	25 mmHg	0.73
9-19.	25 mmHg	0.80
9-20.	299 mmHg	0.33

Required FIO_2

9-21. 36%
9-22. 60%
9-23. 28%
9-24. 19% (but don't use less than 21%)
9-25. 40%

Resultant PaO_2

9-26.	106 mmHg	9-29.	89 mmHg
9-27.	81 mmHg	9-30.	149 mmHg
9-28.	227 mmHg		

Dissolved O_2 Content

9-31.	0.12 mL/dL	9-34.	0.75 mL/dL
9-32.	0.21 mL/dL	9-35.	1.65 mL/dL
9-33.	0.45 mL/dL		

Hemoglobin O_2 Content

9-36.	16.884 mL/dL	9-39.	12.73 mL/dL
9-37.	13.936 mL/dL	9-40.	10.72 mL/dL
9-38.	12.06 mL/dL		

Total O$_2$ Content

9-41. 19.767 mL/dL
9-42. 19.104 mL/dL
9-43. 15.195 mL/dL
9-44. 18.21 mL/dL

9-45. 9.828 mL/dL
9-46. 8.179 mL/dL
9-47. 15.64 mL/dL

Oxyhemoglobin Curve Shift

9-52. L
9-53. R
9-54. R

9-55. L
9-56. L
9-57. R

9-58. R
9-59. L
9-60. N

Oxygen Delivery

9-61. 990 mL/min
9-62. 1146 mL/min
9-63. 608 mL/min
9-64. 728 mL/min

9-65. 686 mL/min
9-66. 820 mL/min
9-67. 1404 mL/min

VO$_2$ and OUC

	VO$_2$	OUC
9-68.	350 mL/min	0.25
9-69.	300 mL/min	0.33
9-70.	300 mL/min	0.18
9-71.	240 mL/min	0.46
9-72.	1050 mL/min	0.35

ABG Interpretation

9-73. Partially compensated metabolic acidosis (acidemia) with adequate oxygenation on room air. Note that although the respiratory system is at or near maximum compensation, the disorder is only partially compensated. This disorder could occur in a patient with diabetic ketoacidosis. It is possible to have an elevated PaO$_2$ on room air when PaCO$_2$ values are low. (Calculate the PAO$_2$ to verify.)

9-74. Partially compensated respiratory acidosis with mild hypoxemia on 30% oxygen. This disorder could occur in a patient with chronic lung disease who is having an acute exacerbation. Maybe his "normal" ABG is pH = 7.37, PaCO$_2$ = 60 mmHg, HCO$_3$ = 31 mEq/L, and PaO$_2$ = 75 mmHg.

9-75. Uncompensated respiratory alkalosis with adequate oxygenation on room air. This disorder could occur in a patient who is afraid of being stuck with a needle.

9-76. Partially compensated metabolic acidosis with moderate hypoxemia on 40% oxygen. This disorder could occur in a patient who is experiencing hypoxemia. The acidemia is occurring because of lack of oxygen (lactic acid production), and the acidemia is stimulating the respiratory center to increase ventilation.

9-77. This blood gas is impossible. There are two acid factors (CO$_2$ of 44 and BE of –3) yet the pH is alkaline. This cannot occur. Someone made a mistake in writing down the values. Also, the PaO$_2$ cannot be 120 mmHg on room air when the CO$_2$ is 44 mmHg.

9-78. Is this a fully compensated metabolic alkalosis, a fully compensated respiratory acidosis, or a mixed defect (a combined respiratory acidosis and metabolic alkalosis)? It is often difficult to interpret such gases without knowing the history of the patient.

9-79. This appears to be a partially compensated metabolic alkalosis with hyperoxemia on 100% oxygen. Actually, this is a post-code patient who responded better than anticipated. He was given much more sodium bicarbonate than should have been given and is now on a ventilator with permissive hypercapnea to keep his pH in an acceptable range until the extra bicarbonate can be eliminated.

9-80. This appears to be a partially (fully) compensated metabolic alkalosis with severe hypoxemia on 24% oxygen. Actually, this is a patient with COPD who is "hyperventilating" owing to the hypoxemia. His "normal" blood gas is pH = 7.35, PaCO$_2$ = 67 mmHg, HCO$_3$ = 38, and PaO$_2$ = 65 mmHg. A partially compensated respiratory acidosis.

Critical Thinking

9-81. Arterial: All values "look" arterial, and the PO$_2$ of venous blood would not be that high. Rare exceptions might include cyanide poisoning or an arterial to venous shunt.

9-82. Arterial: Even though the values are looking a little more like venous values, it would still be rare that a venous blood sample would have a PO$_2$ of 55 mmHg.

9-83. This sample could be venous or it could be arterial. How can it be determined which it is? Color will not help. An arterial sample lying beside a venous sample, both with these values, would look the same. The values themselves will not help either. How quickly the sample filled the syringe might help since venous is a low-pressure system and arterial is a high-pressure system. However, this patient had a low blood pressure. The best thing to do is to look at your patient. If he looks good the sample is probably venous, if he looks bad it is probably arterial.

9-84. Could be arterial or venous. Same reasons as above. Even though the pH seems a bit high for venous and the CO$_2$ a bit low, it could still be venous. Maybe the patient's arterial pH is 7.47 and his CO$_2$ is 20 mmHg.

9-85. Solve this question by performing the following:

$$CaO_2 = 0.003 \times 600 + 1.34 \times 1.0 \times 14;$$
$$CaO_2 = 1.8 + 18.76 = 20.56 \text{ mL/dL}$$

Normally the a-v diff is 5 mL/dL; so . . . , $20.56 - 5 = 15.56$ mL/dL; 15.56 mL of oxygen will be in the venous blood. Since most all oxygen is carried on the Hb, let's do a calculation assuming all oxygen *is* found there.

$$CvO_2 = 1.34 \times O_2Sat \times Hb;$$
$$15.56 = 1.34 \times O_2Sat \times 14;$$

$$O_2Sat = 15.56/(1.34 \times 14);$$
$$O_2Sat = 83\%$$

If the venous blood has an O_2Sat of 83%, the venous PO_2 would be approximately 50 mmHg, even with a PaO_2 of 600 mmHg.

CHAPTER 10

10-1. Reference Table 10-1 in *Respiratory Care*
10-2. Reference Table 10-2 in *Respiratory Care*
10-3. Reference Table 10-3 in *Respiratory Care*
10-4. Reference Table 10-3 in *Respiratory Care*
10-5. Reference Table 10-5 in *Respiratory Care*

Review Questions

10-6. C	10-8. A	10-10. C
10-7. D	10-9. B	10-11. C

CHAPTER 11

11-1. D	11-5. A	11-8. D
11-2. C	11-6. D	11-9. A
11-3. B	11-7. C	11-10. D
11-4. C		

CHAPTER 12

12-2. a. 60 mmHg   e. 93 mmHg
       b. 45 mmHg   f. 52 mmHg
       c. 40 mmHg   g. 68 mmHg
       d. 27 mmHg

12-3. a. 99%   e. 84%
       b. 98%   f. 80%
       c. 96%   g. 55%
       d. 92%

Hemodynamic Parameters

12-4. MAP = 93 mmHg
       MPAP = 17 mmHg
       CI = 2.8
       SV = 70 mL
       PVR = 100 dynes-sec/cm^5
       SVR = 1257 dynes-sec/cm^5
12-5. MAP = 107 mmHg
       MPAP = 32 mmHg
       CI = 3.6
       SV = 75 mL
       PVR = 151 dynes-sec/cm^5
       SVR = 862 dynes-sec/cm^5

Indirect Calorimetry

12-6. Estimated REE based on VO_2 = 1739 kcal/day
       Estimated REE based on the VCO_2 = 1590 kcal/day
       REE based on the Weir Equation = 1738 kcal/day
       RQ = 0.8
12-7. REE = 2500 kcal/day
       RQ = 1.02

Mechanics of Ventilation

12-11. Mean Paw (pres vent) = 18.7 cmH$_2$O with auto-PEEP considered
       Mean Paw (pres vent) = 16.5 cmH$_2$O without auto-PEEP considered
       Mean Paw (vol vent) = 14.9 cmH$_2$O with auto-PEEP considered
       Mean Paw (vol vent) = 12.3 cmH$_2$O without auto-PEEP considered
       corrected VT = 720 mL
       Compliance (VT corrected) = 27 mL/cmH$_2$O
       Compliance (VT not corrected) = 30 mL/cmH$_2$O
       RI = 13 cmH$_2$O/L/sec
       RE = 10.7 cmH$_2$O/L/sec with auto-PEEP considered
       RE = 12.7 cmH$_2$O/L/sec without auto-PEEP considered
       W = 0.21 Kg-M
12-12. Mean Paw (pres vent) = 8.4 cmH$_2$O
       Mean Paw (vol vent) = 6.7 cmH$_2$O
       Corrected VT = 556 mL
       Compliance (VT corrected) = 31 mL/cmH$_2$O
       Compliance (VT not corrected) = 33 mL/cmH$_2$O
       RI = 8 cmH$_2$O/L/sec
       RE = 4.3 cmH$_2$O/L/sec
       W = 0.08 Kg-M

Invasive Monitoring

12-13. P_AO_2 = 225 mmHg
$Sc'O_2$ = 98%
$Cc'O_2$ = 19.06 mL oxygen/dL blood
CaO_2 = 18.28 mL oxygen/dL blood
CvO_2 = 13.05 mL oxygen/dL blood
Qs/Qt = 13%
12-14. Qs/Qt = 14.6

Dead Space

12-15. V_D/V_T = 0.325
V_D = 195 mL
12-16. V_D/V_T = 0.5
V_D = 200 mL

12-17. V_D/V_T = 0.4
V_D = 280 mL

Capnography

12-18. a. start of exhalation
b. V_D
c. mixed V_D and V_A
d. V_A
e. end exhalation/start inspiration
f. inspiratory phase
g. start of exhalation, same as point a

Review Questions

12-19. C	12-22. C	12-25. C
12-20. D	12-23. C	12-26. A
12-21. C	12-24. B	12-27. D

CHAPTER 13

Cylinder Volume and Time of Use

	Volume	Time	
13-7.	14 L	3.5 min	
13-8.	336 L	33.6 min	
13-9.	80 L	16 min	
13-10.	288 L	144 min	2 h and 24 min
13-11.	2512 L	418.6 min	approx. 7 h
13-12.	4710 L	1570 min	26 h and 10 min

Tank Pressure

13-13.	498 psig	13-16.	500 psig
13-14.	1274 psig	13-17.	893 psig
13-15.	662 psig		

Clinical Problem Solving

13-18. 8 "G" cylinders
13-19. 38 min
13-22. 172 min
13-23. 146.5 lbs
13-24. 1963 "E" cylinders

Percent Oxygen Calculations

13-48.	60%	13-50.	38%	13-52.	72%
13-49.	60%	13-51.	76%		

Air:Oxygen Ratios

13-53.	25.3:1	13-56.	2.3:1
13-54.	14.8:1	13-57.	0.52:1
13-55.	6.2:1	13-58.	0.23:1

Total Flow

13-59.	40 L/min	13-63.	104 L/min
13-60.	45 L/min	13-64.	39 L/min
13-61.	48 L/min	13-65.	35 L/min
13-62.	55 L/min	13-66.	22 L/min

Reverse "X" Method, Student Exercise

	Blender Setting	Total Flow
13-67.	33%	48 L/min
13-68.	41%	40 L/min
13-69.	40%	32 L/min
13-70.	45%	38 L/min

13-71. 127%—Impossible; you can't deliver a FIO_2 higher than the entrainment setting.

Review Questions

13-72.	C	13-74. D
13-73.	A	13-75. A

CHAPTER 14

14-1.	27.5 in Hg	14-6.	150 mmHg
14-2.	1088.4 cmH₂O	14-7.	510 cmH₂O
14-3.	517 mmHg	14-8.	13.3 kPa
14-4.	1266 cmH₂O	14-9.	9.8 kPa
14-5.	2.42 atms	14-10.	115.5 fsw

P_AO_2 and the O_2 Equivalent

	P_AO_2	O_2 Equiv
14-11.	116 mmHg	23%
14-12.	211 mmHg	37%
14-13.	496 mmHg	77%
14-14.	1053 mmHg	153%
14-15.	686 mmHg	103%
14-16.	876 mmHg	130%
14-17.	419 mmHg	66%

Oxygen Content

14-18.	11.15 mL/dL	14-22.	22.08 mL/dL
14-19.	10.53 mL/dL	14-23.	7.0 mL/dL
14-20.	14.32 mL/dL	14-24.	12.7 mL/dL
14-21.	14.65 mL/dL	14-25.	6.6 mL/dL

Review Questions

14-26.	C	14-29.	A	14-32.	D
14-27.	C	14-30.	D	14-33.	B
14-28.	C	14-31.	B		

CHAPTER 15

Calculation of Water Vapor Content and PH_2O

	WVC	**PH_2O**
15-1.	13.6 mg/L	13.6 mmHg
15-2.	6.8 mg/L	6.5 mmHg
15-3.	6.92 mg/L	6.6 mmHg (approx)
15-4.	13.84 mg/L	13.8 mmHg (approx)
15-5.	21.8 mg/L	22.4 mmHg
15-6.	5.45 mg/L	5.3 mmHg (approx)
15-7.	15.4 mg/L	15.5 mmHg
15-8.	32.9 mg/L	34.7 mmHg (approx)

Calculation of Potential Humidity and RH

	Potential Humidity	**%RH**
15-9.	15.4 mg/L	71
15-10.	19.4 mg/L	31
15-11.	21.8 mg/L	78
15-12.	21.8 mg/L	23
15-13.	30.4 mg/L	49
15-14.	43.9 mg/L	62
15-15.	43.9 mg/L	87

Calculation of RH at Body Temperature

15-21.	25% RH	15-24.	11% RH
15-22.	14% RH	15-25.	34% RH
15-23.	39% RH		

Calculation of Humidity Deficit

15-26.	38.82 mg/L	15-29.	31.74 mg/L
15-27.	33.52 mg/L	15-30.	12.22 mg/L
15-28.	43.9 mg/L		

Review Questions

15-31.	C	15-34.	C	15-37.	D
15-32.	D	15-35.	B	15-38.	B
15-33.	C	15-36.	C		

CHAPTER 16

Percent Solution Calculation

16-1.	1%	16-4.	5%	16-6.	20%
16-2.	1%	16-5.	4%	16-7.	0.5%
16-3.	10%				

Drug Concentration Calculation

16-8.	2.5 mg	16-13.	12.5 g
16-9.	2 mL	16-14.	15 mg
16-10.	2%	16-15.	2.5 mg
16-11.	2.5 g/50 mL	16-16.	2.5 mg each
16-12.	1 g		

Review Questions

16-17.	B	16-22.	A	16-26.	D
16-18.	B	16-23.	D	16-27.	C
16-19.	C	16-24.	C	16-28.	B
16-20.	B	16-25.	A	16-29.	B
16-21.	D				

CHAPTER 17

17-1. Refer to Table 17-6 in *Respiratory Care*.
17-2. Refer to Table 17-7 in *Respiratory Care*.

Review Questions

17-9.	B	17-11.	A	17-13.	C
17-10.	C	17-12.	D		

CHAPTER 18

Review Questions

18-1.	B	18-6.	A	18-10.	A
18-2.	C	18-7.	C	18-11.	B
18-3.	D	18-8.	B	18-12.	C
18-4.	B	18-9.	B	18-13.	A
18-5.	B				

CHAPTER 19

19-8. mouth-to-mouth, mouth-to-face shield, mouth-to-mask, bag-valve-mask, oxygen demand valve-mask
19-9. The NP airway may have entered the nares and slipped into the patient's laryngeal area.

The patient is gagging on it, and the tube needs to be removed. It most likely will need to be removed with forceps through the mouth.

19-10. The EOA is in the trachea and needs to be removed. Bag-mask ventilation could be done, the EOA re-inserted properly, or the patient intubated.

19-11. Left mainstream intubation, R mainstem obstruction, R pneumonectomy, consolidated R lung, R pneumothorax.

19-12. The cuff is torn. It should be removed and a new tube inserted.

19-13. The contacts may be loose, the bulb may be loose, the bulb may be burned out, the batteries may be dead.

19-14. The size of the tube can be determined by WEIGHT—<1 kg use 2.5 mm, 1-2 kg use 3.0 mm, 2-4 kg use 3.5 mm, >4 kg use 4.0 mm; AGE—premie use 2.5 mm, newborn 3.0 to 3.5 mm; Size of End of Little Finger; Size of External Nares; EXPERIENCE.

19-15. Suction the mouth and oral pharynx. Deflate the cuff slowly until a small leak is heard at end inspiration. Either leave it there or inflate with a small amount of volume until the leak disappears. Measure the cuff pressure when able.

19-16. The tube is too small or the trachea is dilated. If a large leak is present, the cuff is probably not pressing on the trachea and the intra-cuff pressure is not being exerted against the tracheal wall.

Suction Catheter Size

19-20. a. 15 (16) Fr
        b. 13.5 (14) Fr
        c. 12 Fr
        d. 10.5 (10) Fr
        e. 9 (8 or 10) Fr
        f. 7.5 (8) Fr
        g. 6 Fr

Review Questions

19-25. thyroid, cricoid, and epiglottis
19-26. cuniforms, corniculates, arytenoids

19-27. D	19-37. D	19-46. B
19-28. A	19-38. C	19-47. C
19-29. C	19-39. B	19-48. D
19-30. C	19-40. A	19-49. B
19-31. B	19-41. C	19-50. C
19-32. B	19-42. D	19-51. A
19-33. D	19-43. C	19-52. D
19-34. D	19-44. C	19-53. C
19-35. C	19-45. B	19-54. C
19-36. D		

CHAPTER 20

20-10. C	20-18. D	20-25. D
20-11. B	20-19. B	20-26. B
20-12. C	20-20. A	20-27. B
20-13. A	20-21. C	20-28. D
20-14. B	20-22. B	20-29. D
20-15. D	20-23. C	20-30. D
20-16. C	20-24. C	20-31. A
20-17. A		

CHAPTER 21

21-1. a. inspiration
       b. change to expiration
       c. expiration
       d. change to inspiration

21-2. a. time
       b. pressure
       c. flow
       d. manual

21-3. The length of time from the beginning of inspiratory flow to the start of expiratory flow, which begins after the inflation hold (inspiratory pause) if applicable. Flow is routinely measured at the endotube.

21-4. a. time
       b. volume
       c. pressure
       d. flow

Volume Calculation

21-11. 1.0 L	21-19. 40 mL
21-12. 0.8 L	21-20. 25 mL
21-13. 0.4 L	21-21. 75 mL
21-14. 1.25 L	21-22. 100 mL
21-15. 0.8 L	21-23. 100 mL
21-16. 0.8 L	21-24. 53 mL
21-17. 1.2 L	21-25. 60 mL
21-18. 0.6 L	

Review Questions

21-27. D	21-33. D	21-38. A
21-28. D	21-34. B	21-39. B
21-29. D	21-35. D	21-40. B
21-30. A	21-36. B	21-41. B
21-31. A	21-37. B	21-42. D
21-32. B		

CHAPTER 22

Ventricular Rate

22-7. a. 214
     b. 167
     c. 125
     d. 88
     e. 75
     f. 63
     g. 58
     h. 52
     i. 45

Cardiac Rhythm Interpretation

22-8. "P" present - normal - rate = 40
QRS present - sometimes normal - rate = 60, irregular
P and QRS related but P absent with funny-looking beats
P-R interval 0.2 sec
Interpretation: sinus bradycardia with multi-focal PVCs

22-9. "P" present - normal - rate = 80
QRS present - normal - rate = 30
P and QRS not related
P-R interval N/A
Interpretation: third-degree heart block with a slow ventricular response

22-10. "P" not present
QRS present - normal - rate = 60 and irregular
P and QRS N/A
P-R interval N/A
Interpretation: atrial fibrillation (A-fib)

22-11. "P" not present
QRS not present
P and QRS N/A
P-R interval N/A
Interpretation: ventricular fibrillation (V-fib)

22-12. "P" present - normal - rate = 60
QRS present - normal - rate = 60
P and QRS related
P-R interval 0.16 sec
Interpretation: normal sinus rhythm (NSR)

22-13. "P" not present
QRS not present
P and QRS N/A
P-R interval N/A
Interpretation: asystole

22-14. "P" present - normal - rate = 60, irregular
QRS present - normal - rate = 60, irregular
P and QRS related
P-R interval 0.16 sec
Interpretation: sinus bradycardia with atrial premature contractions

22-15. "P" present - normal - rate = 60
QRS present - normal - rate = 30
P and QRS related but some Ps do not have a QRS following it

P-R interval 0.16 sec when present
Interpretation: second degree heart block (Mobitz type II) 2:1 ratio

22-16. "P" present - not normal - rate = 300
QRS present - normal - rate = 75
P and QRS related
P-R interval not measured
Interpretation: atrial flutter with a 4:1 ratio

22-17. "P" not present
QRS present - not normal - rate = 180
P and QRS N/A
P-R interval N/A
Interpretation: ventricular tachycardia (V-tach)

22-18. "P" present - normal - rate = 40
QRS present - normal - rate = 40
P and QRS related
P-R interval 0.28 sec
Interpretation: first degree heart block with bradycardia

22-19. "P" present - normal - rate = 90
QRS present - normal - rate = 60
P and QRS related but some Ps do not have QRS
P-R interval changing
Interpretation: second degree heart block, Mobitz type I (Wenkebach)

Matching

22-20. G   Adenosine
     Q   Atropine
     N   Bretylium
     O   Dobutamine
     J   Dopamine
     F   Epinephrine
     B   Lasix
     C   Isuprel
     M   Lidocaine
     L   Magnesium
     I   Morphine
     D   Nitroglycerine
     P   Nitroprusside
     H   Procainamide
     K   Propranolol
     E   Sodium bicarbonate
     A   Verapamil

Review Questions

22-21. C	22-27. A	22-33. D
22-22. D	22-28. D	22-34. A
22-23. A	22-29. B	22-35. C
22-24. C	22-30. A	22-36. C
22-25. B	22-31. D	22-37. A
22-26. D	22-32. B	

CHAPTER 23

23-2. a. team assessment
      b. patient training
      c. psychosocial intervention
      d. exercise
      e. follow-up
23-3. a. psychiatric disturbances
      b. organic brain syndrome
      c. acute congestive heart failure
      d. recent MI
      e. acute cor pulmonale
         also, substance abuse, significant liver dysfunction, metastatic cancer, disabling stroke

23-4. B	23-8. B	23-12. D
23-5. C	23-9. A	23-13. A
23-6. D	23-10. D	23-14. B
23-7. D	23-11. C	23-15. D

CHAPTER 24

24-1. A	24-5. B	24-9. D
24-2. D	24-6. D	24-10. D
24-3. A	24-7. A	24-11. C
24-4. C	24-8. A	

CHAPTER 25

25-1. C	25-9. B	25-16. C
25-2. C	25-10. B	25-17. C
25-3. D	25-11. D	25-18. C
25-4. D	25-12. B	25-19. A
25-5. A	25-13. B	25-20. B
25-6. C	25-14. D	25-21. A
25-7. D	25-15. A	25-22. D
25-8. A		

CHAPTER 26

26-1. D	26-6. C	26-11. B
26-2. C	26-7. B	26-12. C
26-3. A	26-8. D	26-13. C
26-4. C	26-9. A	26-14. C
26-5. B	26-10. D	26-15. D

CHAPTER 27

27-2. C	27-7. C	27-12. B
27-3. B	27-8. D	27-13. D
27-4. A	27-9. C	27-14. D
27-5. C	27-10. B	27-15. B
27-6. B	27-11. A	26-16. C

CHAPTER 28

28-1. B	28-7. C	28-12. C
28-2. D	28-8. C	28-13. A
28-3. D	28-9. B	28-14. B
28-4. A	28-10. B	28-15. D
28-5. C	28-11. C	28-16. A
28-6. A		

CHAPTER 29

29-1. maintaining ventilation, removing CO_2
29-2. coughing, removing secretions, clearing the airways

29-4. C	29-10. B	29-16. C
29-5. B	29-11. B	29-17. B
29-6. C	29-12. C	29-18. D
29-7. D	29-13. B	29-19. D
29-8. A	29-14. D	29-20. B
29-9. C	29-15. A	

CHAPTER 30

30-1. D	30-5. A	30-8. B
30-2. B	30-6. C	30-9. A
30-3. B	30-7. D	30-10. A
30-4. C		

CHAPTER 31

31-1. C	31-6. D	31-11. B
31-2. B	31-7. B	31-12. C
31-3. D	31-8. D	31-13. B
31-4. B	31-9. A	31-14. B
31-5. A	31-10. D	31-15. B

CHAPTER 32

32-1. D	32-6. D	32-10. D
32-2. A	32-7. B	32-11. C
32-3. B	32-8. D	32-12. D
32-4. B	32-9. C	32-13. A
32-5. C		

CHAPTER 33

Answers to case study:

1. ABG interpretation: severe respiratory acidosis, partially compensated, with mild hypoxemia on 2 L/min nasal cannula

2. Why did E.S. have acute RF? There could be several reasons.

   A. The bump on the head could have been more severe than it appeared. This is unlikely since, following a short time on mechanical ventilation, he was alert and awake and had no further complications.

   B. The patient could have received sedation. None was documented.

   C. Elimination of the hypoxic drive. Patients with COPD, who have chronically elevated $PaCO_2$ levels, have a blunted ventilatory response that is normally present when CO_2 levels increase. These individuals, instead, are said to breathe because of a hypoxic drive, ventilation because of low oxygen levels. Historically, it was believed that when patients with COPD breathed increased oxygen levels, their hypoxic drive was blunted. This would lead to reductions in minute ventilation and further increases in carbon dioxide levels. Another very likely reason for the increased carbon dioxide levels in COPD patients given "too much oxygen" is that their ventilation/perfusion $(\dot{V}/\dot{Q})$ matching is changed. Increased levels of oxygen may cause $\dot{V}/\dot{Q}$ mismatch resulting in increased dead space (V_D) and an increased V_D/V_T ratio resulting in increased $PaCO_2$ levels. One or both of these conditions were probably responsible for the ARF of E. S. Although his PaO_2 was only 68 mmHg when measured, it could have been much higher during the night. Remember that E. S. had been on 1 L/min at home but was found to be on 2 L/min at the time when he was unresponsive.

3. What FIO_2 was being delivered by the nasal cannula at 2 L/min? This can be estimated by using the alveolar air equation. BP = 760 mmHg, PH_2O = 47, and $PaCO_2$ = 149 mmHg. Although PAO_2 is unknown, we know that it had to be at least 68 mmHg because that is what the PaO_2 was.

$$PAO_2 = (BP - PH_2O) \times FIO_2 - (PaCO_2 \times 1.25)$$
$$68 = (760 - 47) \times FIO_2 - (149 \times 1.25)$$
$$68 = 713 \times FIO_2 - 186$$
$$254/713 = FIO_2 = 36\%$$

In this situation, the 2 L/min would be equivalent to at least 36% oxygen. This calculation assumes the a/A ratio is one (1). In reality, the a/A ratio was probably much lower than 1.0, so let's recalculate assuming an a/A ratio of 0.5. (If the a/A ratio was 0.5, the PAO_2 would have been 136 mmHg.)

$$136 = 713 \times FIO_2 - 186$$
$$322/713 = FIO_2 = 45\%$$

With this assumption, the 2 L/min is equivalent to 45% oxygen. The actual delivered FIO_2 was most likely somewhere between these two estimates.

4. Why was the O_2Sat at 83%? A PaO_2 of 68 mmHg would normally have an O_2Sat of approximately 95%. The most obvious cause of the lowered saturation is that the pH is much lower than normal and is shifting the oxyhemoglobin dissociation curve to the right.

5. What was the target value for $PaCO_2$ while E.S. was on the ventilator? E.S. had a history of COPD and was most likely a CO_2 retainer since his HCO_3 was 48 mEq/L. A target value would certainly not be 40 mmHg but probably in the 60 to 70 mmHg range.

Review Questions

33-1. D	33-7. A	33-13. D
33-2. C	33-8. C	33-14. D
33-3. C	33-9. A	33-15. C
33-4. C	33-10. B	33-16. A
33-5. A	33-11. B	33-17. B
33-6. B	33-12. B	

CHAPTER 34

34-1. An acute clinical illness characterized by the development of bilateral pulmonary infiltrates on chest radiographs and severe hypoxemia ($PaO_2/FIO_2 < 200$) in the absence of CHF.

34-2. exudative - proliferative - fibrotic

34-3. C	34-6. B	34-9. B
34-4. A	34-7. D	34-10. A
34-5. C	34-8. C	34-11. C

CHAPTER 35

35-1. C	35-5. D	35-9. B
35-2. A	35-6. D	35-10. D
35-3. A	35-7. B	35-11. A
35-4. A	35-8. B	

CHAPTER 36

36-1. B	36-5. C	36-9. D
36-2. B	36-6. D	36-10. B
36-3. D	36-7. A	36-11. A
36-4. D	36-8. D	36-12. D